The # MAGNESIUM SOLUTION
for High Blood Pressure

JAY S. COHEN, MD

SQUAREONE
PUBLISHERS

The information and advice contained in this book are based upon the research and the personal and professional experiences of the author. They are not intended as a substitute for consulting with a health care professional. The publisher and author are not responsible for any adverse effects or consequences resulting from the use of any of the suggestions, preparations, or procedures discussed in this book. All matters pertaining to your physical health should be supervised by a health care professional. It is a sign of wisdom, not cowardice, to seek a second or third opinion.

COVER DESIGNER: Phaedra Mastrocola
IN-HOUSE EDITOR: Amy Tecklenburg
TYPESETTER: Gary A. Rosenberg

Square One Publishers
115 Herricks Road • Garden City Park, NY 11040
516-535-2010 • 877-900-BOOK • www.squareonepublishers.com

Library of Congress Cataloging-in-Publication Data
Cohen, Jay S.
    The magnesium solution for high blood pressure : how to use magnesium to help prevent and relieve hypertension naturally / Jay S. Cohen.
        p. cm.
    Includes bibliographical references and index.
    ISBN 0-7570-0255-2
    1. Hypertension—Treatment—Popular works. 2. Magnesium—Therapeutic use—Popular works. 3. Magnesium deficiency diseases—Complications—Popular works. 4. Magnesium in the body—Popular works. I. Title.
RC685.H8C567   2004
616.1'32—dc22

                                                    2004005766

Copyright © 2004 by Jay S. Cohen, MD

Printed in the United States of America

10   9   8   7   6   5   4   3   2   1

CONTENTS

ACKNOWLEDGMENTS

I have written books before, but none with such a diverse array of people to thank. Among these are the pioneering members of The Erythromelalgia Association including Karl Granat, Milton Lecouter, Steve Yonker, Ray Salza, Lennia Machen, and many, many others who swapped experiences and information with me, and without whose support I would not be well or writing about magnesium today. My deepest thanks in this regard also to the world-class researchers whose knowledge helped germinate my own about erythromelalgia, allowing me to find the magnesium solution: Dr. Jill Belch of Scotland, Dr. Knut Kvernebo of Norway, Dr. Cato Mork of Denmark, Drs. Thomas Rooke and Mark Davis of the Mayo Clinic, and Dr. Haines Ely.

I'd also like to thank the staff of the *Annals of Pharmacotherapy*, especially Stan Lloyd, Pharm. D; Gene Sorkin, Pharm. D; and Lizanne Sawyer-Kubicki, whose interest in my work led to the publication of my article on magnesium in their prestigious journal. And my special thanks to Dr. Donald Rhodes, a podiatrist and brilliant inventor, whose pioneering work in treating reflex sympathetic dystrophy led to my receiving an accurate diagnosis for the first time, without which none of this would have followed.

In my education about magnesium, many names

stand out: Dr. Mildred Seelig, Dr. Burton Altura, Dr. Chris Mende, Dr. Billie Sahley, and the Gordon Research Conferences. My knowledge has also been advanced by many doctors of integrative medicine who have shared with me their experiences in using magnesium for everyday medical disorders, such as high blood pressure and migraine headaches. Among these: Dr. Allan Magaziner, Dr. Ron Hoffman, Dr. Jeffrey Baker, Dr. James Williams, Dr. Julian Whitaker, Dr. Alan Gaby, Dr. Alan Thal, and Dr. Dan Kalish.

My deepest personal thanks to my family and friends for their support during my long illness that helped me keep going and seeking until finding, beyond our wildest hopes and dreams, the magnesium solution. And to my medical friends who provided support and feedback, and who watched in fascination as my symptoms vanished: Dr. Tony Weisenberger; Mary Weisenberger, RN; Dr. Lee Kaplan; Dr. Dennis Cook; Dede Herst, LCSW; and Dr. Roy Kaplan.

I'd like to add a special acknowledgment to the thousands of doctors and other healthcare professionals who are today opening their minds beyond their heavily pharmaceutical-based sources of information and seeking knowledge about biological and natural substances that make sense scientifically and work clinically. As I've written many times, it is irrational to have two systems of medicine: mainstream and alternative. Integrative medicine, which combines the best of both, is the only medicine that makes sense. Toward this end, this book is the first of a series on natural substances and prescription drugs that I am writing to provide objective, accurate information for patients and their healthcare professionals.

PREFACE

It is no exaggeration for me to say that magnesium saved my life. But it is ironic that I am the one saying it, because during my diverse medical career in general medicine, pain research, psychiatry, psychopharmacology, and now clinical pharmacology, my greatest expertise has always been prescription drugs, not natural supplements. Yet, here I am writing about one of the most important natural substances for maintaining optimal health and treating a wide array of medical conditions.

I didn't learn about magnesium in medical school. Few doctors do. I learned about magnesium the hard way, twenty-eight years later. In 1995, I developed a baffling, painful, rare abnormality of the blood flow to my legs. This vascular (blood vessel) disorder with the strange name, erythromelalgia, left me bedridden for more than 3 years. I underwent all kinds of tests until I couldn't cope with being prodded and punctured any more. I tried every treatment imaginable, mainstream and alternative, to control the disorder's vicious symptoms: excessive blood flow, extreme heat, burning pain, severe swelling, and redness worse than the worst sunburn you've ever seen. I tried spinal blocks, intravenous infusions, hypnosis, biofeedback, acupuncture, hyperbaric oxygen therapy, mercury extraction from my teeth, homeopathy and herbal remedies, and many others.

Most of all, I tried prescription drugs—more than 40 of them. Nothing helped at all, not even morphine. Some treatments made me feel worse.

Finally, at the suggestion of a Scottish researcher, Dr. Jill Belch, I tried a group of drugs I never would have considered. Calcium antagonists (calcium channel blockers) are commonly used for vascular conditions such as high blood pressure, but they had also been reported to trigger my disease, and I wanted no part of any drug that could make me worse. I was already at the far, far end of my rope. Yet, Dr. Belch wrote that sometimes calcium antagonists actually helped erythromelalgia. She didn't know why these drugs sometimes helped, and no one would have expected them to do so, but there it was. I was skeptical and scared, but I was also in terrible pain and had no other options, so I obtained a few tablets of diltiazem (Cardizem), split one into fragments, and started with a very tiny amount.

Gradually increasing the dose over the next few days and watching my body's response carefully, I noticed that my intense pain relented a little. Not much, but enough to be significant. When your pain is at level 10 (10 = maximum pain, 0 = no pain), it makes a big difference if it drops just to level 9. I wasn't even taking a quarter pill, but it was enough to help. Finally, finally, something actually helped. I was elated.

My elation was short lived. As I tried to increase the diltiazem to a more effective dose, I developed muscle spasms and overpowering malaise. Unable to raise the diltiazem enough for any consistent benefit, I switched to other drugs in the group: nifedipine (Procardia) and amlodipine (Norvasc). Both drugs provided the same enticing hint of benefit—and similar problems with unbearable side effects. I was very disappointed, yet not entirely surprised. My specific area of medical expertise is medications and their side effects. I have written medical journal articles and books on these issues, established a widely recognized website at www.MedicationSense.com, and have spoken at the highest levels. I knew that calcium antagonists cause side effects that many patients cannot tolerate. I, unfortunately, was one of them. I felt like Moses, given a vision of the promised land after years of desperation, only to be turned back to the desert of my disease.

I was saved by an unlikely source. In those dark days of early 1999, somewhere from the depths of my mind a connection occurred and a question popped into my consciousness: Isn't magnesium a calcium antagonist? I don't know if this idea arose from some bit of information I absorbed long ago or from God, but magnesium is something I cannot ever remember thinking about previously. That changed quickly.

I soon learned that magnesium is an essential element for the normal activity of nerves and blood vessels, the key players in normal vascular functioning. Indeed, magnesium is the body's natural calcium antagonist, and the balance of magnesium and calcium is key to vascular health. And because magnesium is a physiological element that serves hundreds of important functions in the body, it has virtually no side effects at proper doses. The only real challenge with magnesium is getting it into your body, because most products are poorly absorbed and cause diarrhea, just like milk of magnesia. But once I solved this problem and was able to increase my magnesium intake, my pain quickly eased and my disorder gradually faded.

During those difficult years, I had linked up with others like me through the Erythromelalgia Association, the first and only association in the world for this very rare disorder. Soon I became a Board Member and, later, Chairman of the Medical Advisory Committee, which I remain today. As soon as I was certain of my own improvement with magnesium, I informed the other members. Not every member improved with magnesium. Erythromelalgia, like all vascular diseases, is a complex disorder with many underlying causes, so no one treatment works for everyone.

Yet many people, some disabled or bedridden for years, began to improve. Several of them traveled to San Diego to meet me. It was quite a reunion. These were people who, like me, had been severely disabled by erythromelalgia. Yet there we were, meeting face-to-face for the first time after exchanging hundreds of e-mails and scores of telephone calls over the difficult years when we had pooled everything we knew in the hopes of finding something, anything, to relieve the pain of a heretofore untreatable disease. Some people in our organization who were taking magnesium also reported improvements in other vascular conditions. Magnesium could not only help erythromelalgia, but also migraine headaches, high blood pressure, and muscle spasms. This was not entirely surprising because the medical literature contains hundreds of articles on magnesium's importance for normal vascular functioning and for treating vascular disorders such as high blood pressure, migraine headaches, and Raynaud's phenomena.

In February 2002, I published a scientific paper in the *Annals of Pharmacotherapy* on our group's experience with magnesium for treating erythromelalgia. In early 2004, my research was confirmed when pain specialists in Italy reported that magnesium cured an 8-year-old child with disabling erythromelalgia that had not responded to a variety of drugs and medical procedures.

Just after my paper on magnesium was published, I had the privilege of meeting some of the world's top researchers on magnesium. Scientists from all over the world had assembled for five days at a Gordon Research Conference to discuss one topic: magnesium. These were not fringe scientists or alternative advocates, but academics and mainstream practitioners from the most prestigious institutions in the world. I was stunned to see so much brainpower directed toward one simple element, which most doctors know hardly anything about and never consider for treating patients. Indeed, one of the concerns of the experts at this conference was the difficulty in getting information about magnesium into the hands of everyday practitioners. Without the resources of a drug company for advertising, free seminars, and sales representatives carrying studies and samples to doctors' offices, it is very difficult to get independent information into doctors' awareness. The magnesium researchers published their findings in medical journals, but there are hundreds of medical journals, and doctors may read just a few.

Good medical care requires good information. So with my personal experience with magnesium, my knowledge of drugs and their benefits and risks, and my experience as a writer and speaker, I decided to try to bridge the gap. That's why I've written *The Magnesium Solution for High Blood Pressure:* to get the word out so that you and your doctor can consider this basic, essential element that your body needs and that you can use to help prevent or treat high blood pressure.

Most doctors are wary of supplements that come with all kinds of promises and miracle stories. They should be, and so should you. Fortunately, magnesium comes with scientific evidence that dwarfs the evidence presented for many top-selling prescription drugs. In writing this book, I have provided plenty of information based on scientific evidence, because it is such *evidence-based* information that your doctor will respect. The case for magnesium's importance in treating high blood pressure is very convincing. Yet, so few people know about it. By reading this book, you will know about it. And you can then tell other people and your doctors about magnesium, and then gradually we can reduce the ravages of high blood pressure by adding a safe, inexpensive, physiological therapy—magnesium—to the everyday prevention and treatment of this all-too-common, devastating disease.

—Jay S. Cohen, MD

INTRODUCTION

According to the Joint National Committee on the Prevention, Detection, Evaluation, and Treatment of High Blood Pressure—the recognized experts on treating hypertension—"the goal of prevention and management of hypertension is to reduce morbidity and mortality by the least intrusive means possible."

Over 50 million Americans and 800 million people worldwide (20 percent of the adult population) have high blood pressure (hypertension). Nearly 90 percent of us will develop hypertension in our lifetimes. Hypertension is a devastating disease that damages blood vessels, causing heart attacks, strokes, and other cardiovascular diseases. For this reason, many experts consider high blood pressure more dangerous than high cholesterol. Moreover, many of the severe complications of diabetes stem from the high blood pressure that frequently accompanies it. In short, hypertension is one of the most destructive—and most inevitably destructive—diseases of human beings.

The experts on the Joint National Committee quoted above emphasize the importance of using *"the least intrusive means possible"* for treating hypertension, but in fact mainstream medicine relies almost entirely on powerful prescription drugs even when other safer, proven natural methods are all that are needed. This book is about a safe, natural, inexpensive, non-drug method for treating hypertension that has been proven effective scientifically, yet is routinely overlooked by most doctors. This book is about a simple natural element: magnesium.

When considering any treatment, whether a natural substance or a drug, you should consider the evidence. Is it convincing? Does the treatment make sense? Have studies been done? What do experts say? As you will see in this book, the evidence in all of these regards is huge and convincing for magnesium, and the experts recommending magnesium are many, representing both mainstream and alternative medicine from both the academic and clinical wings.

Scientific evidence is important, but as every medical textbook teaches, the ultimate test is how well a treatment works for individual patients. As we have seen again and again in recent years, many promising drugs with outstanding research have proved ineffective for some patients or toxic for others, necessitating disuse or outright withdrawal. Magnesium's safety has been established over six decades. Today, magnesium is commonly used in cardiac care units for heart arrhythmias. It is used intravenously in maternity units to treat the dangerous effects of eclampsia in pregnant women.

The irony is that despite magnesium's long use in these medically high-risk situations and an extensive body of evidence from magnesium research spanning more than half a century, few medical schools teach doctors anything about magnesium's value for everyday conditions like high blood pressure and migraine headaches. As a result, most doctors aren't aware of magnesium's effectiveness for these common, often difficult-to-treat disorders. Yet, magnesium has proven its value not only in studies, but in the offices of doctors who have learned about it. If you go to a conference on integrative medicine and ask the brightest and best doctors about magnesium, they will relate dozens of experiences of using magnesium with excellent results.

My own experience mirrors this. For example, one day at the University of California, San Diego (where I'm on faculty), I got into a conversation with another professor, Fred. Although Fred exercised regularly and was in good shape, he had developed high blood pressure. "I'm eating more vegetables and fruit," Fred told me, "but my doctor still wants me to take medication. I don't want to."

Like many people, Fred was concerned about side effects, which occur frequently with antihypertensive (blood pressure-lowering) drugs. Indeed, studies have shown that half of the people started on antihypertensive drugs quit treatment within a year, most often because of side effects. Most people quit within ninety days. Drugs that affect blood vessels affect many systems of the body, so side effects can be difficult to avoid.

Because of my expertise on medication side effects, many people with hypertension have contacted me over the years asking how to find treatment they can tolerate for this destructive disease. They had tried drug after drug and got reaction after reaction and, finally, reluctantly, quit treatment. This is such a common story. My answer to such questions is reflected in my medical journal articles, books, website (www.MedicationSense.com), and in the lectures I have been asked to give at major medical conferences and the U.S. Food and Drug Administration. My message consistently is about starting medications, including antihypertensive medications, at the very lowest effective doses. These doses are often 50 percent lower than those recommended by the drug companies and prescribed by doctors.

Lower doses cause fewer side effects. Some people are very sensitive to prescription drugs and do not need the strong standard doses recommended by the pharmaceutical industry. Other people need strong drug doses, but that does not mean their bodies are prepared to handle such potent doses from the start. My research demonstrates the effectiveness of these lower doses, many of which were proven effective in the drug companies' own studies, but are not marketed or even mentioned in medication package inserts or the *Physicians' Desk Reference* because drug companies like to keep dosing simple for doctors. Simple dosing translates into better sales. But it does not translate into better treatment or fewer side effects. That is why for most cases of hypertension, I advocate a "start-low go-slow" approach, and my books tell people exactly how to do this. Other experts, especially experts on hypertension, agree with this method.

However, since my own enlightenment about magnesium in 1999, I recommend taking magnesium first. Why start with strong, expensive, side-effect prone drugs when natural substances often work? From the words of Hippocrates to Thomas Edison to thousands of experts today, healing should begin with good nutrition, then natural supplements. If these do not work, then prescription drugs have a definite role. But too often today, the medical system begins with drugs. This is backwards for mild or moderate hypertension. That is why many patients today are seeking other choices, as Fred sought from me.

Fred needed treatment. At times, his blood pressure rose to 170/110 mmHg (mmHg = the unit of measure for the pressure required to raise mercury one millimeter in a sphygmomanometer, or blood pressure gauge). His diastolic pressure was always at least 100. These are high-risk levels. So I told him about magnesium. Fred was very interested. He read the studies I sent him. He got the magnesium supplement I suggested and started to take it, beginning with a low dose and increasing it gradually, as I advised.

Two months later, Fred reported that his blood pressure was normal. "My diastolic is back to 80, and even under stress it doesn't go over 90."

Knowing that Fred had tried many things, I asked, "What helped you the most?"

He replied, "I attribute the improvement to losing some weight and especially to the magnesium."

Fred was pleased. He had achieved his goal without drugs, without side effects, and without the time and expense of repeated medical visits. "My doctor is amazed," he added.

I was not. Since the 1960s, more than 1,000 articles on magnesium have been published in medical journals. The results are clear: Magnesium is essential for normal vascular functioning. Blood vessels require magnesium to operate properly. Deficiencies of magnesium are common and underlie many common disorders today. One of these disorders is hypertension. It is shocking, frankly, how little people know—how little *doctors* know—about this vital mineral.

One of these doctors was my best friend and one of the leading psychopharmacologists—doctors who specialize in the use of psychiatric medications—in America. Dr. Tony Weisenberger had developed high blood pressure over recent years and was taking prescription drugs. After hearing me talk about magnesium for a while, he finally decided to try it. At its highest, Tony's blood pressure had been 135/90 mmHg, which is high. Months later, on magnesium and off prescription drugs, his blood pressure was a very safe 106/60.

Not everyone responds to magnesium this impressively. Magnesium is not a panacea. Prescription drugs are sometimes necessary. Fred's numbers indicate that he may need a low dose of a prescription drug in the future. But why start with powerful, expensive, side-effect prone drugs when safer, natural methods might suffice? And even if prescription drugs are needed, so is magnesium for your blood vessels to function optimally. Besides, with magnesium, you may need fewer drugs or lower doses, both of which can reduce your risk of side effects, and your drug costs.

Adopting magnesium into the mix of antihypertensive therapies should not be difficult. Doctors are already well aware of the importance of another natural element, potassium, and they recommend it regularly to hypertensive patients. Unfortunately, doctors don't know that to obtain potassium's full effects, magnesium is also essential. Or, that when they prescribe diuretics that wash out potassium, magnesium is washed out too, worsening people's magnesium deficiencies and causing more vascular dysfunction in the long run. We must somehow balance doctors' knowledge of pharmacology with an equal knowledge of physiology, so that doctors will have greater awareness and respect for the natural substances the body uses to maintain health.

I have written this book to provide balance to patients' and doctors' awareness of the possibilities. This book provides you and your doctor with all of the information you need to understand why magnesium is essential for helping to prevent and treat high blood pressure, what you can expect from taking magnesium, and how to take it effectively. This is vital information not only because, unlike drugs, magnesium has virtually no side effects at proper amounts, but magnesium also exerts hundreds of other important effects required for the healthy functioning of your cells and body systems. Magnesium is a key player in the normal functioning of nerves, muscles, blood vessels, bones, and the heart. So when you take magnesium, you not only help your blood pressure, but also help every cell and system in your body.

CHAPTER 1

NORMAL VASCULAR FUNCTIONING AND MAGNESIUM

WHAT IS HYPERTENSION AND WHY IS IT SO HARMFUL?

Just as heightened pressure in the pipes of your house causes erosion and premature rupture, high blood pressure (hypertension) causes accelerated wear and tear in the blood vessels of the human body. This can lead to premature heart attacks, heart failure, strokes, kidney damage, and vascular disorders of the limbs.

Yet, some pressure is needed within the blood vessels for pushing the blood through the body. This pressure develops each time the heart beats, which forces a large amount of blood into the blood vessels, thereby exerting pressure on the walls of the arteries throughout the body. The arteries can expand a bit to absorb some of the pressure, but a certain amount of pressure is necessary to keep the blood moving forward. However, too much pressure is destructive to the walls of blood vessels. This is why it is necessary to maintain a blood pressure that is safe.

What is safe? Blood pressure is measured in terms of

two numbers: the systolic pressure and the diastolic pressure. The systolic pressure is the pressure when the heart pumps blood into the arteries, and the diastolic pressure is the lower pressure between heartbeats. For decades, the ideal blood pressure was considered to be 120/80 mmHg, but today lower pressures are considered optimal. A new term, *prehypertension*, was added in 2003 to the official guidelines of the Joint National Committee on the Prevention, Detection, Evaluation, and Treatment of High Blood Pressure. Prehypertension is defined as having a systolic pressure between 120–139 and/or a diastolic pressure between 80–89 mmHg. Outright hypertension is still defined as a systolic pressure of 140 mmHg or higher or a diastolic pressure of 90 mmHg or higher (see Table 1), but excessive wear and tear on the arteries actually begins at lower pressures. According to the Seventh Report of the Joint National Committee, *"The risk of cardiovascular disease, beginning at 115/75 mmHg, doubles with each increment of 20/10 mmHg."*[1]

How serious is the internal wear and tear caused by high blood pressure? *Conn's Current Therapy*, a leading medical reference, describes it this way:

> A 35-year-old man with an arterial pressure of 130/90 will die 4 years earlier than another 35-year-old man with the same medical background but with normal pressure. If his pressure is 140/90, he will die 9 years earlier, and if it's 150/100, he will die 17 years earlier.[2]

Higher blood pressures are even more devastating. So when you consider that 50 million Americans and 800 million people across the world have hypertension, it is apparent that hypertension is one of the most serious health-care problems today.[3] And when you consider that "most people will develop hypertension during their lifetime," as hypertension expert Norman Kaplan, MD, states in his book, *Clinical Hypertension*,[4] then information about magnesium's role in preventing as well as treating hypertension almost certainly applies to you.

BLOOD VESSELS, HYPERTENSION, AND MAGNESIUM

No one knows what causes most cases of hypertension. A small percentage of cases are caused by adrenal tumors, chronic kidney disease, excessive alcohol intake, or the

Table 1 Blood Pressure Classifications*

This table represents the degree of hypertension associated with different blood pressure levels. Note that, except for Stage 2, experts suggest that hypertension should be diagnosed only after at least two elevated blood pressure readings taken during different office visits. If your systolic and diastolic readings fall into different categories, the higher category defines your blood pressure classification. These classifications do not apply if you are taking antihypertensive drugs or are acutely ill.

	Systolic (mmHg)	Diastolic (mmHg)
Normal	less than 120	less than 80
Prehypertension	120–139	80–89
Stage 1 Hypertension	140–159	90–99
Stage 2 Hypertension	160 or higher	100 or higher

*Adapted from: "The Seventh Report of the Joint National Committee on Prevention, Detection, Evaluation, and Treatment of High Blood Pressure."[5]

use of oral contraceptives or other medications. But more than 90 percent of hypertension develops spontaneously, for no apparent reason. The specific mechanisms underlying spontaneous hypertension (or *essential hypertension*, as physicians call it) are not clear, although it is known that both genetic and environmental factors such as smoking, obesity, and dietary deficiencies play important roles.

We do know that blood pressure is controlled by the tiny smooth muscles lining the interior of blood vessels and the nerves that control them. These muscles' ability to dilate or constrict governs the pressure and blood flow to each organ and tissue, thus allowing the body to adapt to various states such as sleep, digestion, or exercise, as well as to external circumstances such as a hot or cold environment. When the muscles throughout the vascular system dilate, blood pressure drops. When the muscles constrict, blood pressure rises. If this constriction occurs continuously, the blood pressure remains abnormally high. This is hypertension.

What influences the relaxing and tightening of the tiny smooth muscles lining the blood vessels? Many factors, but among the foremost is the mineral magnesium. Actually, the balance of magnesium and another mineral, calcium, in and around the muscle cells lining the arteries is a primary determinant of their state of relaxation and constriction. Calcium tends to make muscles constrict, whereas magnesium causes them to relax. Thus, when excess calcium flows into the muscle cells lining the arteries, constriction occurs and blood pressure increases. There is a whole group of drugs, the calcium antagonists (calcium channel blockers), that doctors prescribe to block the flow of calcium into vascular muscle cells and thereby reduce hypertension. In fact, in the year 2000, doctors wrote more than 95 million prescriptions for calcium antagonists including top-sellers amlodipine (Norvasc), nifedipine (Procardia), diltiazem (Cardizem, Tiazac), and others, at a total cost of over $4.5 billion.[6] These drugs are not only costly, but have many side effects such as dizziness, flushing, palpitations, fatigue, nausea, abdominal pain, tiredness, and swollen legs. Side effects like these cause millions of people to quit treatment for their hypertension, just as I quit taking diltiazem, nifedipine, and amlodipine for my erythromelalgia. But quitting treatment for high blood pressure is not wise either, because untreated hypertension leads to heart attacks, strokes, and premature death. There must be a better solution to this problem.

Fortunately, there is—the magnesium solution—and if doctors were better trained about how the body actually works and about natural (instead of pharmacologic) ways of maintaining healthy functioning, they would know about it. Doctors would know that the body uses magnesium, a natural substance, to block constriction of the blood vessels due to calcium. By blocking the influx of calcium into vascular smooth muscle cells, magnesium regulates blood vessel tone. That is why for decades, experts have called magnesium the body's "natural calcium blocker." [7, 8, 9]

In one major textbook on hypertension, the way in which the magnesium-calcium balance regulates blood pressure is described as follows:

There is mounting evidence that external and internal free magnesium regulates calcium entry and participates in controlling arterial tone. . . . Several lines of evidence suggest that magnesium is reduced in hypertension . . .[10]

In short, excess calcium in vascular smooth muscle cells causes constriction of the blood vessels (vasoconstriction). Magnesium is the natural element your body uses to prevent excess calcium from entering these cells and to maintain normal blood pressure. Magnesium is indeed our natural calcium blocker.

Dr. Sherry Rogers, a leading proponent of integrative medicine, has written extensively about magnesium's benefits for disorders caused by abnormal muscle constriction. "In order for a muscle to contract, it needs calcium. In order to relax it needs magnesium."[11] Hypertension is one of the conditions for which Dr. Rogers uses magnesium.

Magnesium is also necessary for the health of the endothelium, the tiny cells that form the thin inner lining of the blood vessels. Endothelial cells play an active role in prompting the smooth muscle cells to constrict or relax by producing substances such as prostacycline, thromboxane, and endothelin. Magnesium increases the endothelium's production of prostacycline, which induces artery relaxation, and it inhibits the production of thromboxane and endothelin, which promotes artery constriction.[12]

Magnesium also directly influences the ability of cells to use potassium, which also induces artery relaxation. Dr. Mildred Seelig, one of the first pioneers of magnesium research, states, "Low potassium, by itself, can bring on high blood pressure. But even adequate potassium intake cannot normalize high blood pressure if magnesium is too low. Without enough magnesium (and potassium) in our bodies, we cannot expect normal blood pressure."[13]

THE PROBLEM WITH THE STANDARD MEDICAL TREATMENT OF HYPERTENSION

With the exception of the common cold, hypertension accounts for more visits to doctors in the United States than any other condition. Most often, the treatment recommended is some type of prescription drug. Sometimes these drugs are necessary, and there is no doubt their ability to lower blood pressure can prevent many of the severe complications of hypertension.

Yet, most people are not keen about taking prescription drugs, because doing so is expensive and time consuming, and side effects occur all too frequently. Indeed, 50 percent of people who seek treatment for hypertension quit treatment within a year, mainly because of side effects.[14, 15, 16] Other people, fearing the adverse reactions, avoid treatment altogether.

Why do side effects occur so often with antihypertensive drugs? One reason is that the doses that drug companies recommend and that doctors prescribe are too strong for many people. As I showed in an article on this topic in the *Archives of Internal Medicine*, the initial doses recommended by the drug companies and prescribed by doctors are often 100 percent higher than the doses recommended by the Joint National Committee on the Prevention, Detection, Evaluation, and Treatment of High Blood Pressure.[17] These higher doses cause side effects that could be avoided with a more gradual, patient-centered approach. Unfortunately, most doctors do not know about these lower, safer, and proven-effective doses of antihypertensive drugs because they are not mentioned in package inserts or the *Physicians' Desk Reference.*[18] So when doctors prescribe antihypertensive drugs at doses that are too strong for many people, and negative reactions inevitably occur, doctors assume that there is no other recourse but for patients to put up with the side effects.

Indeed, sometimes doctors dismiss side effects as minor, but patients do not. Dizziness, drowsiness, weakness, headaches, nausea, constipation, and/or sexual dysfunctions are not minor to a person who has to put up with this day after day. As Dr. William J. Elliott and his colleagues wrote in an article in *Postgraduate Medicine,* "Often, the cure—the lowering of blood pressure—is perceived as being worse than the disease."[19] It is no wonder so many people quit treatment, making them vulnerable to the ravages of hypertension.

Overall, the drug-oriented approach of mainstream medicine to hypertension is inadequate. A report by the Albert Einstein College Of Medicine summed up the current situation this way:

> Hypertension remains one of the leading preventable causes of disability and death in the United States today. Yet only 21% of patients with high blood pressure are under adequate therapeutic control. The statistics show that about half of treated hypertensive patients discontinue their therapy within a year.[20]

Prescription drugs certainly have a role in treating hypertension, but they do not constitute *the least intrusive means possible,* as the Joint National Committee experts recommend. As Dr. Sherry Rogers, a highly respected doctor of integrative medicine, asserts, "Medicine is hooked on medicines. We need to get hooked on finding the biochemical deficits and correcting them."[21]

She's right, especially for people with prehypertension and Stage 1 hypertension, which constitutes the vast majority of people with high blood pressure. Non-drug methods should be tried first because these methods are natural to the body, cause few if any side effects, cost less—and can be highly successful. First among these natural methods should be magnesium.

Nutritional methods should also be tried for another important reason. Doctors do not like to admit this, but even when antihypertensive drugs normalize your blood pressure, your risk of cardiovascular disease is not completely reduced to the level of someone without hypertension. In other words, the current mainstream treatment of hypertension, even when done successfully, does not completely eliminate your increased risk. This raises a question: Why? Why is it that drug therapy does not reduce the increased risk completely? Perhaps because it does not really address the underlying factors that cause hypertension in the first place. Perhaps because prescription drugs do not provide cells with what they actually need. If your grass turns brown, using a synthetic coloring agent may make it green again, but it will not necessarily make the grass healthy. Prescription drugs may lower blood pressure, but they may not heal the nutritional imbalances within the cells.

Among the nutritional therapies for correcting biochemical deficiencies in vascular cells and treating hypertension, magnesium stands first. In his book, *Magnesium*,

Dr. Alan Gaby, one of the pioneers in the alternative medicine movement, writes: "Magnesium deficiency is one of the most common nutritional problems in the industrialized world today." He adds that while no single vitamin or mineral can cure all of the problems people sustain, "nevertheless, magnesium so often makes a difference in our lives that it deserves special attention. For millions of Americans, correcting magnesium deficiency could be one of the most important steps on the road back to health."[22] This is especially true for people with hypertension.

MAGNESIUM—THE ESSENTIAL ELEMENT FOR NORMAL BODY FUNCTIONING

Magnesium is a mineral that is essential for the normal functioning of the human body. Magnesium plays a key role in more than 300 different enzymatic reactions that take place within all of the body's cells. Magnesium is necessary in just about every step of the path by which cells create energy for their many activities.

Magnesium has a relaxing effect on the central nervous system and tempers the actions of the sympathetic nervous system. Magnesium is essential for cells to maintain proper balances of other minerals such as potassium, sodium, and calcium. When cells are deficient in magnesium, this balance is disrupted, and cells lose potassium and are flooded with calcium and sodium.[23] In the smooth muscle cells of the blood vessels, this sets the stage for constriction and elevation of blood pressure.

Magnesium is also necessary for the proper metabolism of zinc, iron, copper, and phosphorus, as well as for calcium, potassium, and sodium. Within cells, magnesium is essential for regulating many biochemical activities, including the proper metabolism of glucose (blood sugar). Magnesium is essential for normal growth, nerve transmission, wound healing, muscle contraction, and the proper conduction of electrical impulses that govern the functioning of the heart. Magnesium is required for the metabolism of essential fatty acids and many vitamins. Magnesium is an essential element in bone formation and bone resiliency, and it helps to prevent kidney stones. In addition, according to Dr. Sherry Rogers, "Magnesium is one mineral that is in just about every single phase of the detox pathway."[24]

One of America's best-known doctors of integrative medicine, Dr. Julian Whitaker, of Newport Beach, California, writes:

> I often refer to magnesium as my favorite mineral, and with good reason. Magnesium has a known therapy effect on the heart and cardiovascular system; is involved in at least 325 enzymatic reactions throughout the body; helps maintain potassium in the cells; and is vitally important to healing wounds, muscular function, sleep, growth, and healthy pregnancy. Research has overwhelmingly demonstrated the critical relationship between low levels of magnesium and cardiovascular disease. So many hypertensive patients could benefit from increased intake of this mineral.[25]

Dr. Rogers calls magnesium "the king of minerals." She writes that magnesium "has solved more 'incurable' and 'mysterious symptoms' than any other mineral I have observed in 31 years."[26]

CHAPTER 2

MAGNESIUM DEFICIENCY AND HIGH BLOOD PRESSURE

THE MOST COMMON MINERAL DEFICIENCY

In 1900, the average American diet provided about 450 milligrams of magnesium a day. In 2000, the average diet provided only 200 to 225 milligrams daily. The U.S. Recommended Daily Allowance (RDA) of magnesium is 320 milligrams for adult women and 420 milligrams for adult men (see Table 2). This means that while most Americans in 1900 were getting adequate dietary magnesium, today as many as 80 percent of Americans are magnesium deficient.[1,2] Similar deficiencies exist in all Western countries. A survey conducted in France in the mid 1990s found that 72 percent of men and 77 percent of women got less than the RDA of magnesium in their diets.[3] Magnesium deficiencies may be even more prevalent if, as some experts state, the RDA of magnesium is too low and the daily intake should actually be 500 milligrams.

There are many reasons that magnesium deficiencies are much more common today, despite the fact that Americans have more varied food choices than their 1900 counterparts. Some of these reasons are:

- Agricultural fertilizers often contain inadequate amounts of magnesium.

- Accelerated growth techniques in the fields reduce the amount of time for magnesium fixation in plants.

- Refining methods often reduce the magnesium content of foods.

- Boiling vegetables causes loss of magnesium.

- Soft drinks and other popular beverages contain large amounts of phosphates, which interfere with magnesium absorption.

- High-fat diets reduce magnesium absorption.

- The increased amount of calcium that Americans get in foods and supplements reduces the absorption and increases the kidney excretion of magnesium (and other minerals).

- Consumption of large amounts of salt, coffee, and/or

Table 2 U.S. Recommended Dietary Allowance (RDA) for Magnesium

Different ages, genders, and situations require different daily allowances of magnesium. Stress may increase the amount needed. Some experts believe these allowances are too low. Note that the amounts listed represent milligrams (mg).

Age	Men	Women	Pregnant	Lactating
14–18	410 mg	360 mg	400 mg	360 mg
19–30	400 mg	310 mg	350 mg	310 mg
31 or older	420 mg	320 mg	360 mg	320 mg

alcohol can interfere with magnesium absorption or cause magnesium loss from the body.

- Some medications cause magnesium loss: diuretics, which are prescribed for hypertension and congestive heart failure; digitalis; antibiotics such as gentamicin and amphotericin; cancer drugs such as cisplatin; and immunosuppressive drugs that are used to prevent the rejection of a transplanted organ following surgery.

- Most people just do not eat enough magnesium-rich foods: green leafy vegetables, legumes, beans, nuts, soybeans and whole soy products, unprocessed cereals, and unrefined grains.

- Many people take multivitamin or multimineral supplements, but these rarely contain enough magnesium to offset dietary deficiencies. Also, the magnesium contained in many supplements is of poor quality and poorly absorbed.

- The processing of most municipal water and bottled water causes their magnesium contents to be very low.

The result is that day after day, year after year, people are getting inadequate amounts of magnesium in their diets and, consequently, magnesium deficiencies are widespread. Yet, magnesium is essential for the normal functioning of cells and body systems, especially the vascular system, so it is not surprising that vascular disorders such as hypertension, migraine headaches, and Raynaud's phenomenon (a condition characterized by excessive constriction of blood vessels in the fingers and toes, causing pain and spasm in cold environments) affect more than 75 million Americans and approximately 1 billion people worldwide. This is why, of all the nutritional and non-drug methods that people can adopt to prevent and treat hypertension, magnesium supplementation ranks first. Yet, few people—and fewer doctors—know this.

THE EVIDENCE LINKING MAGNESIUM AND HYPERTENSION

There is considerable evidence that links magnesium deficiency with hypertension in humans. Epidemiologic studies (studies of the causes, prevalence, and distribution of disease in population groups) have found a clear, inverse relationship between magnesium in the diet and blood pressure. Specifically, the higher the amount of magnesium in the diets of specific populations, the lower the blood pressure of these populations tends to be; and the lower the amounts of magnesium in the diets of specific populations, the higher the blood pressure of such people tends to be.[4]

For example, in studies of natives of Greenland, the Bantu peoples of southern Africa, Bedouin peoples of the Middle East, and Australian aborigines, the incidences of high blood pressure and cardiac disease were low in these areas where the water or diets were rich in magnesium. When these people moved to urban areas and adopted modern, magnesium-deficient diets, they developed hypertension and cardiac disease as often as Westerners.[5]

Another link that researchers have made between hypertension and magnesium deficiencies is that the incidence of cardiovascular disease is significantly lower in people living in areas with hard water that contains high concentrations of magnesium.[6] Dietary studies also suggest a link between magnesium and blood pressure. Vegetarians, who usually get a lot of magnesium in comparison to non-vegetarians, have a correspondingly lower incidence of hypertension, heart disease, and sudden cardiac death.

The link between magnesium and blood pressure was first recognized in 1925, but little research followed. In 1952, Mildred Seelig, MD, who was then working at Lederle Laboratories (a pharmaceutical company), was amazed to find that antihypertensive drugs worked better in people whose magnesium levels were normal instead of low. Intrigued, Dr. Seelig began doing research on magnesium and its role in health and disease. Over fifty years later, she continues to do so. A former president of the American College of Nutrition, Dr. Seelig has published nearly 100 scientific articles as well as 6 books on magnesium. "There is a clear link between magnesium deficiencies and hypertension," Dr. Seelig told me.[7]

In 1961, Drs. Burton and Bella Altura, working at the State University of New York Health Science Center at Brooklyn, noticed that if vascular smooth muscle was deficient in magnesium, the tiny muscles went into spasm. The contraction could be relieved by replenishing magnesium. "In 1961, everybody was investigating calcium," Burton Altura told me. "We wondered why no one was looking at magnesium. So we decided to include magnesium in our tests. We were so surprised and excited by our findings, we did not believe it. We waited five or six years, repeating our tests hundreds of times, before trying to publish anything."[8]

For over four decades, the Alturas have conducted more studies on magnesium's actions in the body and its role in more medical conditions, including hypertension, than any other research group. In a 1995 article in *Scientific American*, they stated, "At least 10 independent clinical studies show that patients with hypertension of diverse etiologies exhibit hypomagnesemia [low magnesium] in serum or tissues, or both."[9]

Other studies published in the medical literature support the Alturas' conclusions. Below is a sampling of such research. Note that most of these are double-blind, placebo-controlled studies, in which one group of subjects received magnesium, while a comparable group received a dummy (placebo) pill, but neither the researchers nor the subjects knew which people fell into which group. This method is used because it eliminates the possibility of bias by ensuring that the researchers treat all subjects the same way, and the responses of participants themselves are not influenced by psychological factors. For this reason, double-blind, placebo-controlled studies are considered the "gold standard" for valid scientific evidence in medical research and, therefore, trusted by doctors. Such "evidence-based" information is the cornerstone of modern medical treatment. Thus, you may find that your doctor is much more open to the possibility of using magnesium for your hypertension if you show him or her the following study summaries.

• A study published in the journal *Hypertension* in 1989 found that taking 625 milligrams of magnesium daily produced significant reductions in blood pressure in 21 subjects. The authors wrote: "We concluded that appropriate oral magnesium intake might be effective as a nonpharmacological [nondrug] treatment for essential hypertension."[10]

- A study published in the *American Journal of Hypertension* in 1993 found that taking supplemental magnesium produced an average reduction in systolic blood pressure from 154 mmHg to 146, and in diastolic blood pressure from 100 to 92 mmHg in subjects. The authors commented: "For the first time in a double-blind placebo-control study, we have demonstrated that oral magnesium results in a significant dose-dependent reduction of the systolic and diastolic blood pressure."[11]

- A study published in the *International Journal of Cardiology* in 1996 found that taking 600 milligrams of magnesium daily reduced systolic blood pressure by 7.6 mmHg and diastolic pressure by 3.8 mmHg, on average. The authors concluded: "Our results showed that oral magnesium supplementation administered during 3 weeks significantly reduced blood pressure."[12]

- In another double-blind, placebo-controlled study, published in the *British Journal of Nutrition* in 1997, subjects who took 411 to 548 milligrams of magnesium daily experienced a reduction in systolic and diastolic blood pressure.[13]

These and other studies[14, 15, 16] create a compelling body of evidence for the use of magnesium in preventing and treating hypertension. Indeed, the collected evidence is now so strong that in 2001 the U.S. National Institutes of Health stated the following:

Evidence suggests that magnesium may play an important role in regulating blood pressure. . . .The evidence is strong enough that the Joint National Committee on Prevention, Detection, Evaluation, and Treatment of High Blood Pressure recommends maintaining an adequate magnesium intake as a positive lifestyle modification for preventing and managing high blood pressure.[17]

It must be said, however, that not every study on magnesium for hypertension has shown positive results, usually because the studies were too brief for the magnesium to reach maximum effect, or used types of magnesium that were poorly absorbed. Several studies used inadequate doses of magnesium, doses that were even below the recommended daily allowance. If you have a magnesium deficiency, taking the RDA of magnesium will not rectify the deficit and, therefore, have little effect on your blood pressure. Nevertheless, some subjects who received the RDA or even lower doses of magnesium did benefit in these studies, although not enough to achieve statistical significance.

In contrast, the great majority of studies that used higher daily doses of 500 to 1,000 milligrams of magnesium produced statistically significant positive results. In her book *The Magnesium Factor*, Dr. Mildred Seelig reviewed the studies of magnesium for high blood pressure and reached the same conclusion: "The studies that employed the larger supplements of magnesium did in fact show that it has ability to lower high blood pressure."[18]

This is consistent with my experience. In a survey that the Erythromelalgia Association conducted among members who benefited from magnesium, we found that only a few people improved from taking RDA doses, while most—including me—needed 600 milligrams of magnesium daily or more.

THE IMPORTANCE OF MAGNESIUM FOR PEOPLE TAKING ANTIHYPERTENSIVE DRUGS

What if you are already taking medication for high blood pressure? Can magnesium help you? The answer is yes. Magnesium can make the difference between the successful treatment of hypertension or problems in obtaining adequate reduction, help with the difficulties of medications' side effects, or help maintain the proper balance of potassium or other minerals.

Judy, a friend of mine, was having great difficulty with her antihypertensive drugs. Her doctor had prescribed a diuretic and a calcium channel blocker, but the drugs made her feel tired. Worse, Judy was a fitness instructor, and the calcium channel blocker made her muscles tight and caused spasms. I suggested that she switch to magnesium supplements, because magnesium provides the same calcium-blocking effect, yet relaxes rather than tightens muscles. I told Judy to run this idea by her doctor, who agreed to try it. With magnesium and the diuretic, Judy's blood pressure returned to normal, and the muscle spasms and other medication side effects disappeared.

Judy's response is not unusual. Medical studies show that supplemental magnesium can enhance the effects of antihypertensive drugs.[19,20,21] For example, in a 1983 study, twenty subjects who were already taking diuretics were given 375 milligrams of magnesium daily. The magnesium produced substantial additional reductions in both systolic and diastolic blood pressure, and six of the participants were able to reduce the dosage of their drugs. The doctors concluded: "These results indicate that treatment with magnesium should be considered in arterial hypertension at least as an additional treatment in patients already receiving diuretics."[22]

Magnesium supplementation is particularly important for the millions of people who take diuretics such as hydrochlorothiazide, or HCTZ, which is one of the most prescribed drugs in America and found in many generic and brand-name products, including Aldactazide, Dyazide, Esidrix, Hydrodiuril, Maxzide, and Oretic. Other diuretics include chlorthalidone (Hygroton, Thalitone), furosemide (Lasix, Myrosemide), and ethacrynic acid (Edecrin). Diuretics work by inducing the kidneys to excrete sodium, which induces the excretion of excess water. This reduces the volume of fluid in the circulatory system, thereby reducing the pressure. However, diuretics also cause the kidneys to excrete potassium and magnesium.[23,24,25] Doctors know that it is imperative to maintain adequate potassium levels, so they often have patients take potassium supplements or eat potassium-rich foods like bananas. However, most doctors do not know that diuretics also wash out magnesium, or that the body cannot use potassium optimally without adequate stores of magnesium.

In addition, a magnesium deficiency can counteract the effects of antihypertensive drugs. This was recognized decades ago, as Drs. M.P. Ryan and H.R. Brady wrote in the *Annals of Clinical Research* in 1984: "There is evidence that magnesium deficiency may induce resistance to the effects of anti-hypertensive agents."[26] In his book *Magnesium*, Dr. Alan Gaby adds, "The blood pressure-lowering effect of diuretics often diminishes with time because more and more magnesium and potassium are lost. This tends to push the blood pressure back up."[27]

Yet, magnesium depletion usually is not diagnosed, and the magnesium deficiency caused by diuretics is not corrected. Instead, doctors keep upping the doses of anti-hypertensive drugs, which increases the problem of side effects. This is the reason that millions of people quit treatment, leaving themselves vulnerable to premature heart attacks, strokes, and other circulatory diseases. The cost to them and their families, as well as to the economy and healthcare system, is enormous.

Both diuretics and beta-blockers (another class of drugs commonly prescribed for hypertension) can also cause elevations in levels of blood cholesterol, triglycerides, or glucose. All of these effects are unhealthy, especially for cardiovascular health. Augmenting the use of these drugs with magnesium can help keep antihypertensive drug doses low.

Magnesium is particularly important for people with congestive heart failure. In congestive heart failure, the heart becomes less and less able to pump enough blood outward to meet the needs of the rest of the body. This condition often causes weakness, fatigue, shortness of breath, and accumulation of fluid in the extremities, especially the lower legs. In people who have congestive heart failure, cardiac arrhythmias (abnormal heart rhythms) are common and can be rapidly life-threatening. Doctors often prescribe diuretics for people with this condition to reduce the fluid retention and, therefore, the burden on the heart. But if diuretics cause magnesium depletion, the risk of arrhythmias actually increases. Because magnesium has anti-arrhythmia effects, maintaining adequate body stores of magnesium is essential. But as with hypertension, many doctors are not aware of the vital role of magnesium in congestive heart failure, so magnesium deficiencies go unnoticed and uncorrected.

Further, many people with congestive heart failure take digoxin (sold as a generic or brand-name Lanoxin) or other digitalis-type drugs. These drugs can be life-saving, but their use can lead to digitalis toxicity if the drug rises to too high a concentration in the blood. This is a dangerous and all-too-common problem. Symptoms of digitalis toxicity include nausea, loss of appetite, unusual changes in vision, and heart palpitations and irregular pulse. Digitalis toxicity is often associated with magnesium deficiency. Christian W. Mende, MD, a highly respected hypertension specialist, says, "Magnesium deficiency by itself can cause digoxin toxicity, although the digoxin level is normal. This is well known with potassium deficiency, but not appreciated with magnesium deficiency."[28]

THE FAILURE TO
IDENTIFY MAGNESIUM DEFICIENCY

According to Dr. Robert Whang:

> Magnesium depletion may represent the most frequently unrecognized electrolyte abnormality in clinical practice today. . . . There appears to be as much as an 85 to 90 percent shortfall in clinical recognition of abnormal serum magnesium. . . . The role of magnesium in cellular function, both in health and disease, remains largely unknown to [medical] clinicians.[29]

The fact that humans can become deficient in magnesium was not discovered until 1956. Yet, in the years since, only a small portion of the mainstream medical community and the general public has become aware of the prevalence of magnesium deficiency and its impact on health. Why? The training of most medical doctors does not focus on magnesium. If doctors do not know about magnesium deficiencies, they cannot diagnose them or teach others about them. So, although a small, dedicated group of researchers around the world continues to conduct studies and hold conferences, spreading the word has been difficult. This is not likely to change without funding from the National Institutes of Health or a foundation to subsidize the effort.

"Physicians are a lot less knowledgeable about magnesium than [they are about] calcium," Dr. Mende has told me. "More studies on magnesium such as by the National Institutes of Health are needed for prevention and treatment of magnesium-related diseases. Research on magnesium could have as major an impact on public health as many other items the NIH is studying."[30]

The main reason that magnesium deficiency is not widely recognized is the lack of a readily available, reliable test for the condition. Today, most medical laboratories measure the total serum (blood) magnesium. This usually is not helpful because even if a person is severely deficient in magnesium, the body keeps the blood level normal by pulling magnesium out of cells and bone. A person can have a major magnesium deficiency, yet still have a serum magnesium level that is normal. Incidentally, the same is true for calcium; thus osteoporosis is not diagnosed by a blood test, but by measuring bone density.

For decades, scientists have searched for a simple test to identify magnesium deficiencies. This has not been easy because less than 1 percent of the body's total magnesium is contained in the blood, whereas about 55 percent resides in bone, 26 percent in muscles, and 18 percent in the other tissues. Developing a test that accurately reflects magnesium levels in tissues has been a challenge.

The traditional test for measuring magnesium deficiencies is the magnesium-loading test. Two grams of magnesium are injected intravenously or intramuscularly (a potentially painful process) and patients must collect their urine over the next 24 hours. This is not wildly popular among patients. Yet, the test is highly accurate, because people with adequate magnesium stores in their body will excrete most of the injected magnesium. People without adequate magnesium will excrete only a small portion. The standard is that people who excrete more than 80 percent of the injected magnesium are not magnesium deficient, whereas people who excrete less than 80 percent are magnesium deficient. However, some people are genetically unable to retain magnesium, even when they are severely deficient. Thus, with the magnesium-loading test, these people will excrete most of the injected magnesium, and their test results will be read as normal, whereas in fact they have severe magnesium deficiencies.

More recently, Drs. Burton and Bella Altura and others have developed a test that measures the ionized (electrically charged) fraction of magnesium in the blood, rather than measuring the total serum magnesium. They call it the IMg2+ test. They report, "We have found that even borderline hypertensives usually exhibit significantly depressed serum ionized, but not total, magnesium levels. By measuring ionized magnesium levels by our methods, we find that among patients with untreated hypertension with systolic pressures above 140 or diastolic pressures above 90, 70 to 80 percent have low magnesium levels."[31] This is an astonishing finding that, if confirmed, could change medicine's entire approach to hypertension. However, this test is not widely available yet, although it can be obtained by contacting: Drs. Burton and Bella Altura, Department of Physiology—Box 31, SUNY Health Service Center at Brooklyn, 450 Clarkson Avenue, Brooklyn, NY 11203-2056.

Another reliable test, known commercially as Exatest, measures the total magnesium taken from a swab of cells from your inner cheek or under your tongue. The laboratory, Intracellular Diagnostics, will send a kit to your doctor, who will smear the cells onto a slide. The laboratory uses energy-dispersive analysis to measure the level of magnesium and other minerals within the cells. This test is usually covered by Medicare and other insurers. Check with Intracellular Diagnostics Inc., 553 Pilgrim Drive #B, Foster City, CA 94404. Tel: 650-349-5233. Website: www.exatest.com.

Doctors who practice integrative medicine sometimes also use a test that measures the level of free magnesium in red blood cells. This test is available through the laboratories used by the individual practitioners.

These new tests offer promising possibilities. Yet, the fact is that until an accurate magnesium test is as accessible and covered by insurance as other blood tests, magnesium deficiencies will continue to go undiagnosed and untreated. The fault for this lies not only with the absence of a convenient test, but first and foremost with inadequate medical education and medical practices that are overly wedded to the drug industry—which spends billions to keep doctors focused on prescription drugs, not natural substances. Doctors who are aware of the importance of magnesium for maintaining health and treating vascular diseases find ways around today's limitations in magnesium testing. Some doctors order the tests listed above. On the other hand, Dr. Mende uses the standard magnesium blood test at his disposal, which is inexpensive, although not highly accurate at identifying people with magnesium deficiencies. "Still, I catch many patients with low magnesium," Dr. Mende states.[32] He prescribes magnesium not only for people identified as having low magnesium levels, but also for those with magnesium levels in the bottom third of the normal range.

This is not a bad approach. Experts believe that the "normal range" of the total serum magnesium test is so broad that almost everyone falls into it, yet people whose levels are in the lower end of the normal range are probably magnesium deficient. For the most accurate results, the test should be taken fasting (in the morning before eating), and the result must be adjusted if the level of serum albumin (a type of blood protein) is abnormal. Even with these imprecise guidelines, the total serum magnesium test can identify many magnesium deficiencies.

Nevertheless, if you or your doctor has access to more accurate tests, you should use them. When these more precise methods become readily available, testing for magnesium will become as routine as testing people's calcium levels. The result will be a much greater recognition of magnesium deficiency, a truly widespread problem. Then, treatment with magnesium—which is safe, effective, and inexpensive—might finally become a standard for preventing and treating high blood pressure, as well as migraine headaches, Raynaud's phenomenon, and other cardiovascular disorders.

CHAPTER 3

MAGNESIUM DEFICIENCIES IN HIGH-RISK POPULATIONS

OLDER ADULTS, HYPERTENSION, AND MAGNESIUM DEFICIENCIES

Even in healthy people, blood pressure tends to rise with age. In people between the ages of eighteen and forty-nine, only about 4 percent develop hypertension. But by the time people reach the ages of seventy to seventy-nine, nearly two-thirds have high blood pressure (see Table 3).

In 1950, only 8 percent of the American population was age sixty-five or older. By 1990, the proportion had increased to 12.5 percent, and by 2040 it will be around 20 percent. And as the population gets older, the proportion with hypertension will rise even higher.

By the time a person reaches the age of sixty, diastolic pressure (the second number in the blood pressure measurement) has usually peaked. In fact, it often decreases a bit after age sixty. In contrast, systolic pressure (the first number) usually continues to rise until the eighth or ninth decade of life. The presence of a rising systolic pressure combined with a level diastolic pressure leads to a form of hypertension called *isolated systolic hypertension* or ISH.

Isolated systolic hypertension is the most common form of hypertension in people over age sixty-five. You have ISH if your systolic pressure is 160 mmHg or higher and your diastolic pressure is 90 mmHg or lower. A systolic pressure between 140 and 159 mmHg, coupled with a diastolic of 90 or less, is considered borderline ISH.

Recognizing and treating ISH is important because, according to hypertension authority Dr. Norman M. Kaplan, "In the elderly, systolic pressures are better pre-

Table 3 The Incidence of Hypertension Increases With Age

The following table indicates the prevalence of hypertension, by age, in the general population in the United States, as measured in surveys between 1988 and 1991. Note that in these surveys, hypertension was defined as having a systolic pressure of 140 mmHg or higher and/or a diastolic pressure of 90 mmHg or higher, or already taking antihypertensive medication.*

Age Group (in years)	Percentage With Hypertension
18–29	4 percent
30–39	11 percent
40–49	21 percent
50–59	44 percent
60–69	54 percent
70–79	64 percent
80 or over	65 percent

*Centers for Disease Control, National Center for Health Statistics, Third National Health and Nutrition Examination Survey, 1988–1991.

dictors of cardiovascular risk than are diastolic pressures."[1] Isolated systolic hypertension is usually treated just like any other form of hypertension. This usually means the use of diuretics, because they are effective, inexpensive, and usually well-tolerated, but as we have seen, diuretics have the undesirable effect of washing out magnesium and potassium. Doctors usually take care to replace potassium in people taking diuretics, but most doctors are not aware of the effects of diuretics on magnesium, so they rarely recommend replacing it, too. Doctors routinely check potassium blood levels in older people taking diuretics and potassium supplementation; they should order magnesium blood levels as well.

WOMEN, HYPERTENSION, AND MAGNESIUM DEFICIENCIES

Over thirty million American women have hypertension. Hypertension is the most common risk factor for cardiovascular disease, and heart disease and strokes are the number-one and number-three causes of death in American women.[2] High blood pressure is less common in younger women than it is in younger men, but it is more common in older women than in older men. After age sixty-five, hypertensive women outnumber men with high blood pressure, and more hypertension-related deaths occur in women.

According to Dr. Norman Kaplan, "The development of hypertension in women is associated with increasing body weight, alcohol consumption, and less high-fiber food—and magnesium intake."[3] Dr. Kaplan bases this statement on a study of more than 40,000 women published in 1996. After observing the women for many years and then analyzing the factors that might have contributed to the development of hypertension, the study identified low intakes of magnesium and fiber as having a significant association with elevated blood pressure. No other minerals—not sodium, not potassium, not calcium—were linked to the blood pressure elevations. The researchers concluded, "The inverse association between magnesium and blood pressure in our study suggests that intake of this mineral may play a role in blood pressure regulation."[4]

A 1994 study supported this conclusion. In this double-blind, placebo-controlled study, 91 middle-aged and older women took 500 milligrams of magnesium daily. Both systolic and diastolic pressures were reduced in the magnesium group. The researchers stated, "The findings suggest that oral supplementation with magnesium may lower blood pressure in subjects with mild to moderate hypertension."[5]

Other factors also play a role in high blood pressure for women. More middle-aged women than men are overweight, and obesity is a demonstrated risk factor for developing hypertension. Also, women are now routinely told to take calcium to prevent osteoporosis, but calcium supplementation can block magnesium absorption and increase magnesium excretion, worsening magnesium deficiencies. Magnesium is also important for bone health, but unfortunately, magnesium supplementation is rarely suggested by healthcare professionals.

Among younger women, birth control pills are a common cause of elevated blood pressure. About 5 percent of women who take oral contraceptives develop hypertension, with women who are in their mid-30s or older having the greatest risk. Adequate intake of magnesium and potassium, coupled with weight control and exercise, might help reduce this risk.

Women also frequently run in to problems when prescribed medications for high blood pressure. Most antihypertensive drugs are prescribed at the same doses for a 250-pound man and a 110-pound woman. Many women have difficulty tolerating these strong doses and develop side effects. This is an even greater problem for women age sixty or older, who constitute 60 percent of this age group. These older women are typically treated with the same strong drug doses that are prescribed to young men, even if the older woman has other medical conditions and takes multiple medications. Avoiding medication side effects means tailoring drug doses to individual needs and tolerances, but this is rarely done in today's rushed medical environment. (For information about how medication dosages can be properly adjusted for people of different sizes, ages, genders, states of health, and degrees of medication sensitivity, please consult my articles published in the medical literature[6,7,8] or my book, *Over Dose: The Case Against The Drug Companies* (Tarcher/Putnam 2001), which contains chapters specifically on women, the elderly, and how to use antihypertensive medications safely.[9])

AFRICAN-AMERICANS, HYPERTENSION, AND MAGNESIUM DEFICIENCIES

Hypertension is more prevalent among African-Americans than among Caucasians. Blacks and whites demonstrate similar blood pressures in childhood, but blood pressures are generally higher in adults of African ancestry than in those of European descent. This difference increases with age, so that, overall, black men and women have nearly twice the incidence of hypertension than white men and women do. A number of different explanations have been proposed for this, including stress, genetics, and socioeconomic factors such as diet.

Mineral metabolism is also a factor in such increased incidences of high blood pressure for this group. It is widely recognized that African-Americans retain sodium more than people of other ethnic backgrounds, and African-Americans demonstrate greater elevations in blood pressure when they consume salt. Because of this heightened salt sensitivity, salt restriction is usually a basic component of the treatment of African-Americans who have hypertension.

Yet another mineral may also be involved. In a study published in 1997, Dr. Lawrence M. Resnick and colleagues at the Cardiovascular Center of the New York Hospital-Cornell Medical Center detected "the presence among hypertensives and among black subjects (independently of blood pressure) of a consistent depletion of circulating magnesium and of an imbalance of calcium and magnesium that may potentiate vascular disease among these subjects."[10] In other words, the levels of magnesium, as measured by the ionized magnesium test, were low in African-American subjects whether or not they had hypertension. This coincides with the findings from a 1995 study: "The results showed that serum magnesium levels and dietary magnesium intake were both lower in blacks than whites."[11]

Because hypertension is so widespread in the African-American community, treating it is considered an urgent health-care issue. Yet hypertension in African-Americans is more resistant to standard medical treatment than it is in whites. The wide prevalence of magnesium deficiencies in the African-American population may explain this resistance. If magnesium deficiencies are more widespread and more severe among blacks, their poorer responses to standard antihypertensive drugs should not be surprising. Therefore, magnesium supplementation may be particularly important for African-Americans with hypertension.

DIABETES, HYPERTENSION, AND MAGNESIUM DEFICIENCIES

People with diabetes have a three- to five-fold greater risk of dying from cardiovascular disease than non-diabetics. One of the main reasons for this is that people with diabetes are much more likely to develop hypertension. Statistics vary somewhat, but it is clear that 40 to 80 percent of people with diabetes ultimately develop hypertension. The result is that today more than 11 million Americans have both diabetes and hypertension.

This is a dangerous combination. Both diabetes and hypertension cause vascular damage leading to heart disease, stroke, and kidney failure, but this damage is greatly accelerated when diabetes and hypertension exist together. According to an article published in the December 2001 issue of the *Archives of Internal Medicine*, "Hypertension can contribute as much as 75% of all diabetes mellitus-related complications."[12]

An article titled "A New Message Emerges in Treating Diabetes," published in the *New York Times* in September 2003, stated:

Studies show that cardiovascular disease, set off mainly by hypertension, is the leading cause of death among people with diabetes, and two of every three diabetes-related deaths are caused by heart disease or stroke. . . . Many experts believe that lowering blood pressure may be the most important step—even more important than reducing blood sugar—that people with diabetes can take.[13]

Yet, a survey by the American Diabetes Association showed that 68 percent of people with diabetes were not aware of this risk. And you can bet that far more are unaware of the central role that magnesium plays in the connection between diabetes and hypertension. In an article published in *Diabetes Care* in 1995, endocrinologist Zachary T. Bloomgarden, MD, reported, "Studies have shown that 90 percent of individuals with type 2 diabetes [non-insulin dependent] have low levels of free intracellular red blood cell magnesium."[14] In 1997, Dr. Lawrence Resnick concluded that "a link between magnesium, diabetes mellitus, and hypertension seems established beyond a reasonable doubt." He added, "The lower the free magnesium [the level of magnesium circulating freely in the bloodstream], the stiffer the blood vessels, the higher the blood pressure, the greater the insulin resistance."[15]

In 2001, the U.S. National Institutes of Health described why magnesium is so important for diabetics and why these individuals' magnesium levels are usually low:

Magnesium is important to carbohydrate metabolism. It may influence the release and activity of

insulin, the hormone that helps control blood glucose levels. Elevated blood glucose levels increase
the loss of magnesium in the urine, which in turn
lowers blood levels [of] magnesium. This explains
why low blood levels of magnesium are seen in
poorly controlled type 1 and type 2 diabetes.[16]

This would also explain the link between diabetes, low
magnesium, and high blood pressure.

Magnesium plays other vital roles in the health of
diabetics. Magnesium is necessary for maintaining adequate potassium, which is also essential for maintaining normal blood pressure. Magnesium may be essential
for controlling diabetes itself. In *Scientific American*, re-
nowned magnesium researchers Drs. Burton and Bella
Altura wrote, "Data scattered in the literature collective-
ly suggests that control of diabetes is inversely related to
magnesium deficiency." That is, the difficulty in controlling diabetes is directly related to increasing severities of
magnesium deficiencies. The Alturas continued:

Diabetic retinopathy [eye damage due to diabetes]
is clearly associated with a state of magnesium
deficiency. We thus propose that magnesium deficiency is a characteristic of chronic, stable, mild non-
insulin-dependent diabetes and may predispose
patients to the excess cardiovascular mortality of the
diabetic state.[17]

Recent evidence also suggests that an abnormal balance of calcium and magnesium—too much calcium in
relation to too little magnesium—in the body's tissues
may underlie the development of insulin resistance,

which is the impairment in glucose metabolism that often precedes diabetes. These findings led the authors of a 2001 article to conclude that this abnormal balance of calcium and magnesium "may be the common cellular pathway that links hypertension, obesity, and non-insulin-dependent diabetes."[18]

Taking oral magnesium supplements has been shown to improve both insulin-dependent diabetes and non-insulin-dependent diabetes.[19,20,21] Yet, although magnesium deficiencies in hypertension and diabetes were demonstrated decades ago, in 2002 the problem still remained largely unrecognized by mainstream physicians. This fact led Dr. Resnick to assert: "The time has thus finally come to translate what is already known of the critical importance of magnesium in cardiovascular function and glucose and insulin metabolism into clinical practice."[22]

ALCOHOL USE, HYPERTENSION, AND MAGNESIUM DEFICIENCIES

Although recent reports suggest that modest alcohol consumption helps prevent coronary heart disease, this does not change the fact that excessive alcohol intake can cause hypertension. According to the American Heart Association, "Alcohol intake of more than 3 drinks per day is associated with approximately a doubling of the prevalence of hypertension."[23] Excess alcohol use also interferes with the effects of antihypertensive drugs.

Research shows that reducing alcohol intake to two or fewer drinks daily reduces blood pressure. For most people, consuming one or two drinks a day has no harmful effects on blood pressure. However, some people, particularly women, may be unusually sensitive to alcohol's impact on blood pressure and need to reduce alcohol intake even further, or not drink alcohol at all.[24]

It now appears that magnesium deficiency is linked to the hypertension that occurs in heavy drinkers. Alcoholics are almost always deficient in magnesium, as well as many other nutrients. Studies have shown that alcoholics have significantly lower magnesium levels within their body's cells than non-alcoholics. Also, alcohol alters the calcium/magnesium balance in cells. [25, 26] Just about every heavy drinker needs magnesium supplementation. Indeed, one of the traditional treatments for people entering alcohol rehabilitation programs is an injection or oral supplementation of magnesium.

CHAPTER 4

How to Use Magnesium to Help Prevent and Treat Hypertension

MAGNESIUM: A NUTRIENT AND A MEDICATION

Whether or not you have a documented magnesium deficiency, magnesium may benefit you. I did not measure my magnesium level before trying it; it never occurred to me to do so. Now, after taking substantial doses of magnesium every day for years, I am certainly not magnesium deficient, but I still need the nutrient. The magnesium keeps my erythromelalgia in remission, and if I discontinue it or reduce the dosage too much, my symptoms start to return. This is because the mineral magnesium has both nutritive and, at higher doses, pharmacologic effects.

Magnesium promotes relaxation of the blood vessels and tones down the sympathetic nervous system. Thus, if a pregnant woman develops eclampsia, a dangerous complication characterized by severe hypertension and a high risk of seizures, her doctor will immediately treat her with large doses of magnesium, administered intravenously. The doctor will not question whether or not the woman has a magnesium deficiency. Magnesium is the standard treatment for this condition because it reduces blood pressure and calms an excited nervous system quickly and safely.

Dr. Allan Magaziner, President of the American College for the Advancement of Medicine, orders tests for magnesium levels for all of his patients with hypertension. Yet, he has told me, "Even if the test is normal, I still use magnesium. Even in people without low magnesium tests, magnesium still has a therapeutic effect. Magnesium is nature's calcium channel blocker. There are hundreds of articles on its use in vascular disease including hypertension, congestive heart failure, coronary spasm, recovery from heart attacks, atrial fibrillation or virtually any other arrhythmia [abnormal heart rhythm]."[1]

Whether or not you have hypertension, you may still have a magnesium deficiency—most people do. Each year, millions of people spend hundreds of dollars for vitamins, minerals, and other supplements even though they have no reason to suspect that they have deficiencies of these substances. However, there is ample reason for anyone to wonder if they have a magnesium deficiency, because such deficiencies are pervasive and most people do not get the recommended levels of magnesium in their daily diets. Magnesium supplementation makes as much sense—perhaps more sense—than taking vitamin C or other supplements every day.

"Like the antioxidants, vitamin E and vitamin C," Dr. Julian Whitaker states, "I have separated out magnesium, because I think of all the elements to supplement, magnesium is the most important. This impoverished second cousin to calcium is routinely ignored by conventional physicians, and I will never understand why."[2]

PREVENTING HYPERTENSION

Preventing hypertension is the number-one goal of hypertension specialists. The Joint National Committee on the Prevention, Detection, Evaluation, and Treatment of High Blood Pressure (the acknowledged experts on hypertension), states:

> Before considering the active treatment of hypertension, the even greater need for prevention of disease should be recognized. A significant portion of cardiovascular disease occurs in people whose blood pressure is above the optimal level (120/80 mmHg) but not so high as to be diagnosed or treated as hypertension.[3]

Keeping blood pressure from rising even to the level of prehypertension (see page 10) is important. According to an article published in the *New England Journal of Medicine* in 1997, the serious health risks from hypertension "increase with progressive elevations in blood pressure, beginning at even normal levels of blood pressure."[4]

Because of the importance of preventing hypertension, the Joint National Committee has recommended a nationwide effort to reduce blood pressure in America. The benefits, as described by the Joint National Committee, would be enormous:

> An effective population-wide strategy to prevent blood pressure rise with age and to reduce overall blood pressure levels, even by a little, could affect

overall cardiovascular morbidity and mortality as much as or more than that of treating only those with established disease.[5]

How might this be accomplished? Their answer is by having people exercise regularly, eat a healthful diet, reduce their salt consumption, and increase their potassium intake. These efforts are very important, but I and other experts would also add magnesium. Indeed, studies have suggested that magnesium's greatest effect may be in preventing hypertension from developing in the first place.[6] If you are concerned about preventing hypertension or have been told that you have high-normal blood pressure, taking the recommended daily allowance of magnesium makes sense. In fact, some experts think the current RDAs are too low and suggest taking 500 milligrams of magnesium daily.[7]

TREATING HYPERTENSION

Dr. Whitaker describes the case of John, a 55-year-old, slightly overweight man with a Stage 2 blood pressure of 160/110 mmHg. John had already been taking diuretic and beta-blocker medications prescribed by his mainstream physician, and his blood pressure had dropped somewhat—but so did his energy level and sex drive. Dr. Whitaker then prescribed a balanced, low-fat diet and a vitamin and mineral regimen that emphasized potassium and magnesium. Dr. Whitaker reports on John's results:

He was soon able to withdraw from both medications and enjoy a normal sex life, as well as normal blood pressure. John's experience is common to many. Most high blood pressure patients who make the dietary changes John was instructed to, particularly supplementation with magnesium and potassium, will experience the same results.[8]

For people with established hypertension, the best results are often achieved with a combination of methods that includes magnesium supplementation. According to hypertension specialist Dr. Christian Mende:

> Increasing magnesium alone will not cure hypertension in many people, but it is one aspect of a comprehensive approach. Hypertension is always multifactorial. It is 60 percent genetic, involving at least twelve genes, and about 40 percent environmental, which includes smoking, obesity, diet, etc. To treat people successfully, you have to address all of the factors. Magnesium deficiency is one common factor that must be addressed.[9]

The majority of people with high blood pressure have mild, Stage 1 disease, but this should not lull anyone into complacency. Dr. Norman M. Kaplan notes that the majority of medical complications of hypertension do not occur "in the relatively few with severe disease, but in the masses of patients with blood pressures that are only minimally elevated."[10] In addition, because the blood pressures of people with hypertension tend to rise even higher over the years, it is very important to start treatment early when the condition can best respond to non-drug methods like magnesium.

Where should you and your doctor start? Here is Dr. Magaziner's approach:

I use magnesium as my first line of treatment. Sometimes I use magnesium alone, sometimes with potassium and fiber. I start with more than one thing if they've had hypertension a long time and if their blood pressure is very high or they are on several antihypertensive drugs. Otherwise, I often start with magnesium alone. I start at 400 mg/day. If necessary, I will increase to 400 mg twice-daily.[11]

Dr. Whitaker sometimes recommends as much as 1,000 milligrams of magnesium per day, combined with 2,000 milligrams of calcium plus potassium.[12] A small percentage of people may respond to the modest recommended daily allowance of magnesium, but in my experience, many people require more. Dr. Seelig recommends starting with 700 milligrams a day of magnesium and, if no result is seen over several weeks, increasing gradually to as high as 1,200 milligrams per day.[13]

Improvement can occur within weeks, but sometimes it takes several months. This is because it is very difficult to force magnesium into cells. In contrast, calcium readily rushes in. Thus, cells must work to get magnesium inside and then use the magnesium to block the entrance of excessive calcium. The process takes time, and people differ in how quickly their cells can assimilate magnesium, and in the degree of their deficiencies. It can take up to a year for serum magnesium levels to rise. For me, magnesium's benefits first became apparent after three weeks, but its maximum effect was not attained for many months.

Even with magnesium and other healthful methods, some people will still require prescription drugs to lower their blood pressure sufficiently. If this is your situation,

then drugs—at the lowest doses necessary—shou
used. Although I prefer non-drug approaches, pres... ....
tion drugs are not the enemy—the enemy is hypertension
and the ravages it wreaks on blood vessels. Used appro-
priately, medications for high blood pressure can help
to prevent strokes, heart attacks, congestive heart failure, kidney damage, and the worsening of hypertension itself. Even alternative doctors agree. Dr. Magaziner
told me:

> I do use prescription drugs. Absolutely. Alternative
> medicine isn't a panacea. That's why it's called 'com-
> plementary,' because you have to use drugs some-
> times, too. But we try to keep them to a minimum;
> generally they are not our first choice. Unfortunate-
> ly, with conventional medicine, if you have a symp-
> tom, you get a prescription drug. The mentality is
> that prescribing a drug is the only thing you can do,
> yet this simply is not the case.[14]

If you need prescription drugs for hypertension, the
dose can usually be kept lower if you also use magnesium, potassium, and other non-drug methods as well.
Less medication means fewer side effects, lower costs,
and fewer long-term risks. Based on recent studies, many
experts recommend a diuretic as the first drug for treating hypertension.[15] But diuretics, which work by causing
the kidneys to eliminate more fluids and reduce the volume of blood and thereby the pressure in the vascular
system, also wash out potassium and magnesium. So getting enough of these two vital, blood pressure-lowering
minerals is vital for people taking diuretics. Potassium
can be replenished by eating vegetables or fruit, but it is

difficult to get enough magnesium from foods. This is why supplementation is often necessary.

Some antihypertensive drugs do not cause losses of magnesium and potassium. The popular angiotensin-converting enzyme (ACE) inhibitors, for example, work by blocking the production of angiotensin, a hormone that causes blood vessels to constrict. When diuretics are needed, some doctors prescribe combination drugs such as Dyazide or Aldactazide; or generic equivalents that contain hydrochlorothiazide (HCTZ), a diuretic; and either triamterene or spironolactone, which are drugs that prevent potassium and magnesium loss. Amiloride (Midamor), combined with HCTZ in Moduretic, also spares potassium and magnesium. But if you are already magnesium deficient, these drugs may not be enough to correct the deficiency. Magnesium supplements may still be necessary, but if you are also taking a drug designed to prevent the loss of magnesium and potassium, supplements should be started at low doses and monitored by your doctor.

Doctors often try to offset the mineral losses caused by diuretics by prescribing potassium supplements, but rarely recommend magnesium supplements too. Potassium supplementation is only partially helpful, because it does nothing to offset the magnesium deficiencies caused or worsened by the drugs. The mineral deficiency, in turn, hinders potassium use by the cells.[16] "Magnesium deficiency keeps people from replenishing potassium," Dr. Mende says. "So when patients are hospitalized and potassium levels are low, efforts to increase potassium often are hampered—unless the magnesium deficiency is also treated."[17]

Indeed, having patients take potassium and calcium supplements without including magnesium can cause additional problems. "Potassium and calcium loading of the patient with undiagnosed magnesium inadequacy is not only often unsuccessful, but it may carry inherent risks," state Dr. Mildred Seelig and Dr. J.P. Sheehan. "It can intensify the magnesium depletion, the arterial contractility, and electrocardiogram abnormality."[18] Magnesium supplementation is essential.

TYPES OF MAGNESIUM SUPPLEMENTS

Using magnesium successfully depends on finding a product that agrees with you. Some people can take any product, but many people have difficulty with magnesium, especially cheap, low-quality products that are poorly absorbed. When you take magnesium tablets or capsules, your body absorbs only about 30 percent of the magnesium they contain. With many top-selling products, absorption is much less, as little as 10 percent. This is because minerals like magnesium—or calcium or iron—are the stuff of rocks, and the human body is not designed to absorb rocks. When magnesium is not absorbed, it goes to the colon and can cause gas or diarrhea. This is why Milk of Magnesium, which is intentionally formulated to be poorly absorbed, works very well as a laxative. Poor-quality magnesium supplements can have the same effect. Therefore, the type of magnesium you choose can be very important.

You cannot purchase magnesium in its pure form, because atomic magnesium, like most elements, has an electric charge and readily binds with other atoms in nature. That is why there are so many different types of

magnesium supplements available: magnesium carbon-
ate, magnesium oxide, magnesium chloride, magnesium
sulfate, and others. For better absorption, some supplement companies combine magnesium with amino acids,
producing magnesium maleate, magnesium citrate, magnesium lactate, or magnesium aspartate, which work
well for many people.

When I developed erythromelalgia, I did not know
much about magnesium, and I had great difficulty tolerating many supplements. My gut did not like any of
them, not even the amino-acid complexes. I almost gave
up, but finally found a type of magnesium that worked
well: magnesium chelate, which is an organic complex of
magnesium with amino acids and proteins. This is the
type I recommend for people who have trouble with
other types of magnesium, or who want to avoid the possibility of developing trouble. I also suggest magnesium
chelate for people whose physicians recommend higher
doses of magnesium for their medical conditions. Many
vitamin and health food stores carry chelated supplements, or they can order some for you. You can also find
many sources of magnesium chelate on the Internet.

My experience is that for people with vascular conditions, magnesium products that do not contain other
minerals work better than combination formulas. Even
for nutritional purposes, I prefer taking a separate magnesium supplement because many calcium-magnesium
or other combination products contain poor-quality
types of magnesium that are poorly absorbed.

If you have difficulty with magnesium pills, you may
do better with a liquid solution, particularly magnesium
chloride solution. Magnesium solutions cost more than

tablets or capsules, but they are the best absorbed, best tolerated, and fastest acting forms of the mineral. Some vitamin and health food stores carry magnesium-only solutions or dissolvable powders, but these products can be hard to find on shelves. However, stores can usually special-order liquid magnesium for you, or you can find it online. Overall, I prefer magnesium pills because they are less expensive and more convenient to use, and their effects last longer throughout the day. But if you cannot tolerate them, liquid magnesium is for you. And because liquids are absorbed faster, liquid magnesium is ideal for acute vascular conditions such as acute migraines.

HOW MUCH MAGNESIUM TO TAKE

Because individual responses to magnesium vary, I recommend starting at a lower dose than the recommended daily allowance (see page 21) and increasing gradually. For example, you might start by taking 100 milligrams of magnesium once or twice a day. Over a week or two, you can increase it to the RDA (320 mg/day for women, 420 mg/day for men). You should be sure to get plenty of fluids because the body eliminates excess magnesium through the kidneys. It is best to take magnesium supplements with meals, as this improves absorption.

For medical conditions, people often have to use magnesium doses that are well above the RDA level. This should be done with medical supervision. If you are an older adult, have kidney impairment, or are taking drugs that can affect blood pressure, you should have your doctor supervise the use of even the recommended daily allowance of magnesium. If magnesium causes gas or loose stools, discontinue until it stops, then proceed again more gradually or switch to another type of magnesium supplement. It is not unusual to go through a little trial and error to find what works best for you. For the long-term, you should take calcium and other minerals in balance with the magnesium.

Unfortunately, getting your doctor's cooperation may be your greatest hurdle. Most doctors know little about magnesium. That is why I have written this book like an evidence-based medical journal article—the type of scientific paper that doctors respect. If you show your doctor this book and he or she still will not help, there are many other people you can turn to. Many other healthcare professionals—doctors who practice integrative medicine, nutritionists, naturopaths, nurses, chiropractors, and others—usually know about magnesium and can guide you.

Major problems with magnesium are rare. In 2000, an international journal stated, "The therapeutic window [the range of safe doses] of magnesium is wide, and in the absence of renal failure, severe side effects are extremely rare."[19] The rare case of magnesium toxicity that does arise usually occurs in a person with kidney impairments, or in older people whose kidney functioning is reduced.

If you accidentally take more magnesium than your body can use or eliminate, the first symptoms you might experience include nausea, weakness, feeling of warmth, or flushing. Low blood pressure, reduced heart rate, double vision, and slurred speech can also occur. Like any mineral when taken at extremely high doses, severe magnesium toxicity can be dangerous; it can cause extreme weakness, vomiting, loss of reflexes, respiratory and/or cardiac arrest. Magnesium toxicity can be diagnosed by means of a blood test; total serum magnesium, which most medical laboratories perform, will reveal an elevated magnesium blood level. Magnesium toxicity is worsened by low calcium levels. Calcium gluconate is an effective antidote.

DIETS FOR HYPERTENSION AND THE ROLE OF MAGNESIUM

If you have Stage 1 or Stage 2 hypertension and your doctor is eager to prescribe medication for you, remind him or her that experts recommend trying three to six months of non-drug treatment first. As one leading textbook states, "Because of its low risk profile, non-pharmacologic therapy must always be considered the cornerstone of blood pressure treatment."[20]

In fact, as researchers probe the genetic origins of hypertension and develop newer and better drugs to treat the condition, we are rediscovering that diet is much more important than usually recognized. Yet many Americans do not eat a healthy diet, and according to a 2001 report, "In persons with established hypertension or at risk of developing hypertension, diet quality is even worse [than average]."[21]

Hypertension can often be prevented or improved with a reasonably good diet. "Some people still need medicines and there is a place for them," states Dr. Barry Elson, an expert in integrative medicine, "but I would venture to say that most patients on antihypertensive medicine will not need it if they have the proper lifestyle and nutrient support."[22] Mainstream medicine agrees. The Joint National Committee on the Prevention, Detection, Evaluation, and Treatment of High Blood Pressure says, "Even when lifestyle modifications alone are not adequate in controlling hypertension, they may reduce the number and dosage of antihypertensive drugs needed to manage the condition."[23]

What are the elements of good nutrition for preventing or treating hypertension? If you are overweight, losing weight is the single most important step you can take. The problem is that, although most people know this, more than 62 percent of Americans are overweight and the number continues to rise. Telling them to lose weight is a tough sell.

Many cases of hypertension are caused by an improper mineral balance in the body.[24] This can be corrected by adopting the Dietary Approaches to Stop Hypertension (DASH) diet. This diet does not require reducing either calories or salt. In clinical trials, the DASH diet reduced systolic blood pressure by 11.4 mmHg and diastolic pressure by 5.5 mmHg, on average, in people with Stage 1 hypertension.[25] These reductions equal the reductions achieved with many antihypertensive drugs.

Why does the DASH diet work? Because it restores the proper balance among magnesium, potassium, sodium, and calcium in the body. How important is the mineral rebalancing that is accomplished with the DASH diet? It is estimated that if all Americans adopted the DASH diet, as many as 225,000 heart attacks and 100,000 strokes would be *prevented each year*. Modest salt restriction would improve these results even further.[26]

The DASH diet includes fish, poultry, fruits, vegetables, whole grains, low-fat dairy products, and nuts. As compared with the typical American diet, it contains reduced amounts of fats, red meats, sweets, and sugar.[27] The DASH diet works mainly because it provides large amounts of magnesium (about 500 milligrams a day) and potassium, as well as calcium. The amount of magnesium is key. This was confirmed in a 1995 study from the Netherlands, which demonstrated magnesium's primary role above other minerals in lowering blood pressure: "The relation between magnesium intake and blood pressure was stronger than those between blood pressure and intakes of potassium and calcium."[28] Furthermore, in his 1997 article, Dr. Lawrence Resnick of the Wayne State University Medical Center stated: "Magnesium intake is an independent predictor of blood pressure and of the prevalence of hypertension in large populations—often more significantly related to disease risk than other mineral elements such as sodium and calcium."[29]

The bottom line is this: Eating the right diet—with enough magnesium, potassium, and calcium—provides major benefits for people with hypertension. Moreover, healthy diets like the DASH diet reduce cholesterol and triglyceride levels, improve glucose metabolism and bone integrity, and lower the risk of cardiovascular disease, diabetes, and some cancers.

Experts agree that the best source of minerals and other beneficial nutrients is a good diet. However, even with a healthy diet, getting enough magnesium is not easy. Nuts and legumes, which contain large amounts of magnesium, are also high in calories, which can negate efforts to lose weight. Other foods that contain magnesium include beans, sweet potatoes, tofu, spinach and other leafy green vegetables, broccoli, cauliflower, cheese, shellfish, whole-grain breads, cereal, red meat, and rice. Yet even with these varied food sources, getting just the recommended daily allowance of magnesium is difficult. Thus, many people need magnesium supplementation.

SODIUM, POTASSIUM, CALCIUM, AND OTHER NON-DRUG METHODS FOR REDUCING HIGH BLOOD PRESSURE

Many people are under the impression that restricting sodium intake reduces blood pressure. This is not always the case, but it works often enough to make it worth giving it a try. The average American gets more than 3,600 milligrams of sodium daily, the equivalent of about 9 grams of table salt. Medical experts recommend reducing this intake to 2,400 mg, about 6 grams of table salt. [30] Because many people get 75 percent of their sodium from processed foods, reading labels and requesting reduced salt at restaurants can make a big difference.

Reducing salt consumption is not as effective at lowering blood pressure if you are also deficient in potassium. Indeed, for people with hypertension, getting enough potassium may be more important than reducing sodium. Potassium reduces both blood pressure and cardiovascular risk. Dr. Julian Whitaker states:

> Potassium by itself acts like a diuretic by ridding the body of excess sodium and fluid. I have noted that when my patients with normal blood pressure eat a diet rich in potassium and magnesium and low in salt, the rings on their fingers become looser as they begin to shed water and sodium.[31]

One easy, effective way to improve your body's mineral balance is by switching to a table salt that contains a combination of sodium, potassium, and magnesium instead of standard sodium chloride. A 1984 study of people who were already taking medication for hypertension found that switching from regular salt to a combination salt reduced blood pressure and lowered blood glucose levels. [32] More recently, studies employing sodium-potassium-magnesium mixtures (in an 8:6:1 ratio) as a cooking and table salt produced significant reductions in both systolic and diastolic blood pressures.[33,34] These mineral mixtures are available at food markets or health food stores.

Although the direct effect of calcium on lowering blood pressure is small, calcium reduces the body's sensitivity to the hypertensive effects of sodium. Without adequate calcium, sodium pushes blood pressure higher. Other nutrients and supplements that can lower blood pressure modestly include: vitamin C, alpha lipoic acid, vitamin E, arginine, vitamin B_6 (pyrodoxine), coenzyme Q_{10}, garlic, and hawthorn.

In addition to these, the evidence for the positive effects of omega-3 oils (fish oils) is quite strong. Regular exercise also reduces blood pressure and protects against cardiovascular disease. However, if you are over thirty-five and/or have been sedentary for some time, you should get your doctor's approval before beginning any new exercise regimen. Also, start gradually and work up to longer or more strenuous workouts, being careful not to overdo it.

CONCLUSION

Consider these two related problems:

- Eight hundred million people worldwide, including 50 million Americans, have high blood pressure. Two million Americans are newly diagnosed with hypertension each year, as the Joint National Committee reports. Yet, a third of Americans with hypertension do not know they have it, and most people with hypertension do not receive adequate treatment.

- Seventy-five percent of people in industrialized Western countries are magnesium deficient. The great majority of these people are not aware that they are deficient in magnesium.

There is a connection between these two facts. Hypertension occurs when blood vessels lose their flexibility and become rigid. Excess calcium in the smooth muscles lining the blood vessels causes them to become rigid. Magnesium, which is the body's natural calcium blocker, keeps excess calcium from entering these cells. By doing so, magnesium relaxes blood vessels, reduces blood pressure, and enhances the beneficial effects of potassium, which most doctors know is important in maintaining normal blood pressure. In other words, having an adequate amount of magnesium allows blood vessels (and other muscles of the body) to operate optimally.

Unfortunately, magnesium deficiencies are rampant—and so is hypertension. To me, the connection is obvious, and the evidence is compelling.

Despite this, very few doctors know anything about magnesium's vital role in normal body functioning. Doctors rarely diagnose magnesium deficiencies, order magnesium tests, or recommend magnesium supplementation. Indeed, doctors frequently prescribe drugs that cause or worsen magnesium deficiencies, although they are not aware of the fact. This is a major problem.

Nevertheless, for tens of millions of people, magnesium is the key. This simple mineral can help prevent hypertension. Magnesium can help bring mild hypertension back to normal levels and enhance the effects of weight loss and exercise. For people with severe hypertension, magnesium can help restore normal blood vessel functioning and reduce the amount of drugs needed to keep blood pressure under control. Less medication means fewer side effects, less likelihood of discontinuing treatment, and reduced risks of the heart attacks, strokes, and other diseases that result from hypertension.

However, magnesium is not a panacea. Magnesium alone will not cure all cases of hypertension. Just like with medications and just about everything else in life, people can respond very differently to magnesium. In one study, 40 percent of the subjects taking magnesium obtained blood pressure reductions of 10 mmHg or more, while others obtained more moderate reductions, and others obtained little blood pressure reduction. Moreover, although the mineral's benefits can often be seen quickly, its full benefits usually take time to build as the body gradually moves more magnesium into the cells.

Although I saw improvement in my erythromelalgia, it took several months to reach maximum benefit.

Our drug-oriented healthcare system is not very good at spreading the word about proven-effective, natural alternatives like magnesium. The big marketing money is channeled into advertising expensive drugs that produce huge profits. These profits are directed into producing more drugs and advertising them vigorously to the public and, especially, to doctors. Because so much money is spent on marketing highly profitable prescription products, natural supplements—including those backed by substantial scientific evidence—get overshadowed. Prescription drugs deserve an important role in treating hypertension, but are not always the leading role. Medical experts (such as the Joint National Committee) recommend using *the least intrusive means possible* when treating hypertension, especially in initial treatment. Magnesium is far less intrusive than prescription drugs; it is the very element that the body employs to maintain blood vessels' flexibility.

If you have high blood pressure, you should obtain a medical evaluation and proper diagnosis. If you need treatment, remember that the initial treatment of Stage 1 and 2 hypertension, as well as prehypertension, should be *non-drug* methods. These should be tried for several months. Non-drug methods include weight loss, exercise, a balanced diet, smoking cessation (if you smoke), stress reduction—and magnesium supplementation. Magnesium is a natural element, easily available, safe, inexpensive, essential for normal body functioning, imperative for normal blood vessel functioning—and proven effective in helping to prevent and treat hypertension.

REFERENCES

1. Normal Vascular Functioning and Magnesium

1. Chobanian, A.R., Bakris, G.L., Black, H.R., et al. "The seventh report of the Joint National Committee on prevention, detection, evaluating, and treating high blood pressure." *JAMA*, 2003; 289:2560–2571.

2. Rakel, R.E. *Conn's Current Therapy*. Philadelphia: W.B. Saunders Company, 1993.

3. Chobanian, A.V. "Control of Hypertension—an Important National Priority." *New England Journal of Medicine*, 2001; 345(7):534–35.

4. Kaplan, N.M. "Hypertension in the Population at Large." Chapter 1 in *Clinical Hypertension*. Baltimore: Williams and Wilkins, 1998.

5. Chobanian, A.R., Bakris, G.L., Black, H.R., et al. "The seventh report of the Joint National Committee on prevention, detection, evaluating, and treating high blood pressure." *JAMA*, 2003; 289:2560–2571.

6. Latner, A.W. "34th Annual Top 200 Drugs." *Pharmacy Times*, 2000; 66(4): 16–32.

7. Rude, R.D. "Magnesium deficiency: a cause of heterogeneous disease in humans." *Journal of Bone and Mineral Research*, 1998; 13(4):749–58.

8. Iseri, L.T., and French, J.H. "Magnesium: nature's physiologic calcium blocker." *American Heart Journal*, 1984; 108(1):188–93.

9. Altura, B.M., and Altura, B.T. "Role of Magnesium in the Pathogenesis of Hypertension Updated." Chapter 72 in Laragh, J.H., Brenner, B.M., *Hypertension: Pathophysiology, Diagnosis, and Management*. 2nd Edition. New York: Raven Press Limited, 1995.

10. Swales, J.D. *Textbook of Hypertension*. Oxford: Blackwell Scientific Publications, 1994.

11. Rogers, S.A. *Tired or Toxic? A Blueprint for Health*. Syracuse, New York: Prestige Publishing, 1990.

12. Seelig, M.S., and Rosanoff, A. *The magnesium factor*. New York: Penguin Group Inc. 2003.

13. *Ibid*.

14. Chobanian, A.V. "Control of Hypertension—an Important National Priority." *New England Journal of Medicine*, 2001; 345(7): 534–35.

15. Feldman, R., Bacher, M., Campbell, N., et al. "Adherence to pharmacologic management of hypertension." *Canadian Journal of Public Health*, 1998; 89(5):116–8.

16. Bloom, B.S. "Daily Regimen and Compliance with Treatment." *BMJ*, 2001; 323:647.

17. Cohen, J.S. "Adverse drug effects, compliance, and the initial doses of antihypertensive drugs recommended by the Joint National Community vs. the Physicians' Desk Reference." *Archives of Internal Medicine*, March 26, 2001; 161:880–85.

18. *Physicians' Desk Reference*, 54th–57th Editions. Montvale, NJ: Medical Economics Company, 2000–2003.

19. Elliott, W.J., Maddy, R., Toto, R., Bakris, G. "Hypertension in Patients with Diabetes." *Postgraduate Medicine*, 2000; 107:29–38.

20. Hypertension Management Today, Albert Einstein College Of Medicine, Office Of Continuing Medication, June 1996; 1(1):1–14.

21. Rogers, S.A. *Tired or Toxic? A Blueprint for Health*. Syracuse, New York: Prestige Publishing, 1990.

22. Gaby, A. *Magnesium: How an Important Mineral Helps Prevent Heart Attacks and Relieve Stress*. New Canaan, CT: Keats Publishing, 1994.

23. Rude, R.D. "Magnesium deficiency: a cause of heterogeneous disease in humans." *Journal of Bone and Mineral Research*, 1998; 13(4):749–58.

24. Rogers, S.A. *Tired or Toxic? A Blueprint for Health*. Syracuse, New York: Prestige Publishing, 1990.

25. Whitaker, J. "Miraculous Magnesium, Calcium, and Other Minerals Used against Hypertension." Chapter 6 in *Dr. Whitaker's Hypertension Report—1997*.

26. Rogers, S.A. "Cure for Resistant Magnesium Deficiency." *Total Wellness Newsletter*, Nov. 2001:1–3.

2. Magnesium Deficiency and High Blood Pressure

1. Rogers, S.A. *Tired or Toxic? A Blueprint for Health*. Syracuse, New York: Prestige Publishing, 1990.

2. Johnson, S. "The multifaceted and widespread pathology of magnesium deficiency." *Medical Hypotheses*, 2001; 56(2):163–70.

3. Galan, P., et al. "Dietary magnesium intake in French adult population." In: Theophile, T, Anastassopoulou, J. *Magnesium: current status and new developments*. Dordrecht [Netherlands]: Kluwer Academic, 1997.

4. Altura, B.M., Altura, B.T. "Magnesium in Cardiovascular Biology." *Scientific American*, Science & Medicine, May/June 1995:28–37.

5. *Ibid*.

6. Altura, B.M., Altura, B.T. "Role of Magnesium in the Pathogenesis of Hypertension Updated." Chapter 72 in Laragh, J.H., Brenner, B.M., *Hypertension: Pathophysiology, Diagnosis, and Management*. 2nd Edition. New York: Raven Press Limited, 1995.

7. Seelig, M.S. Personal communication, April 23, 2001.

8. Altura, Burton. Personal communication, Dec. 6, 2001.

9. Altura, B.M., Altura, B.T. "Magnesium in Cardiovascular Biology." *Scientific American*, Science & Medicine, May/June 1995:28–37.

10. Motoyama, T., Sano, H., Fukuzaki, H. "Oral magnesium supplementation in patients with essential hypertension." *Hypertension*, 1989;13(3):227–32.

11. Widman, L., Wester, P.O., Stegmayr, B.K., Wirell, M. "The dose-dependent reduction in blood pressure through administration of

magnesium. A double blind placebo controlled cross-over study." *American Journal of Hypertension*, 1993;6(1):41–5.

12. Sanjuliani, A.F., de Abreu Fagundes, V.G., Francischetti, E.A. "Effects of magnesium on blood pressure and intracellular ion levels of Brazilian hypertensive patients." *International Journal of Cardiology*, 1996:56(2):177–83.

13. Itoh, K., Kawasaka, T., Nakamura, M. "The effects of high oral magnesium supplementation on blood pressure, serum lipids and related variables in apparently healthy Japanese subjects." *British Journal of Nutrition*, 1997;78(5):737–50.

14. Kawano Y., Matsuoka H., Takishita, S., Omae, T. "Effects of magnesium supplementation in hypertensive patients: assessment by office, home, and ambulatory blood pressures." *Hypertension*, 1998;32:260–265.

15. Dyckner, T., Wester, P.O. "Effect of magnesium on blood pressure." *BMJ*, 1983;286(6381):1847–9.

16. Witteman, J.C., Grobbee, D.E., Derkx, F.H., et al. "Reduction of blood pressure with oral magnesium supplementation in women with mild to moderate hypertension." *American Journal of Clinical Nutrition*, 1994;60(1):129–35.

17. Facts about Dietary Supplements. Office of Dietary Supplements, National Institutes of Health, Mar. 2001.

18. Seelig, M.S., Rosanoff, A. *The magnesium factor.* New York: Penguin Group Inc., 2003.

19. Dyckner, T., Wester, P.O. "Effect of magnesium on blood pressure." *BMJ*, 1983;286(6381):1847–9.

20. Saito, K., Hattori, K., Omatsu, et al. "Effects of oral magnesium on blood pressure and red cell sodium transport in patients receiving long-term thiazide diuretics for hypertension." *American Journal of Hypertension*, 1988;1(3 Pt 3):71S-74S.

21. Wirell, M.P., Wester, P.O., Stegmayr, B.G. "Nutritional dose of magnesium in hypertensive patients on beta blockers lowers systolic blood pressure: a double-blind, cross-over study." *Journal of Internal Medicine*, 1994;236(2):189–95.

22. Dyckner, T., Wester, P.O. "Effect of magnesium on blood pressure." *BMJ*, 1983;286(6381):1847–9.

23. *Ibid*.

24. Reyes, A.J., Leary, W.P. "Cardiovascular toxicity of diuretics related to magnesium depletion." *Human Toxicology*, 1984;3(5):351–71.

25. Durlach, J., Durlach, V., Rayssiguier, Y., et al. "Magnesium and blood pressure. II. Clinical studies." *Magnesium Research*, 1992;5(2):147–53.

26. Ryan, M.P., Brady, H.R. "The role of magnesium in the prevention and control of hypertension." *Annals of Clinical Research*, 1984;16 (Suppl 43):81–8.

27. Gaby, A. *Magnesium: How an Important Mineral Helps Prevent Heart Attacks and Relieve Stress*. New Canaan, CT: Keats Publishing, 1994.

28. Mende, C. Personal communication, Sept. 25, 2001.

29. Whang, R. "Chapter 2, Clinical Perturbations in Magnesium Metabolism." In Theophile, T., Anastassopoulou, J. *Magnesium: current status and new developments: theoretical, biological, and medical aspects*. Dordrecht [Netherlands]: Kluwer Academic, 1997.

30. Mende, C. Personal communication, Sept. 25, 2001.

31. Altura, B.M., Altura, B.T. "Magnesium in Cardiovascular Biology." *Scientific American*, Science & Medicine, May/June 1995:28–37.

32. Mende, C. Personal communication, Sept. 25, 2001.

3. Magnesium Deficiencies in High-Risk Populations

1. Kaplan, N.M. "Hypertension in the Population at Large." Chapter 1 in *Clinical Hypertension*. Baltimore: Williams and Wilkins, 1998.

2. Cohen, E., Wheat, M.E., Swiderski, D.M., Charney, P. "Hypertension in Women." Chapter 11 in Laragh, J.H., Brenner, B.M., *Hypertension: Pathophysiology, Diagnosis, and Management*. Second Edition. New York: Raven Press Limited, 1995.

3. Kaplan, N.M. "Hypertension in the Population at Large." Chapter 1 in *Clinical Hypertension*. Baltimore: Williams and Wilkins, 1998.

4. Ascherio, A., Hennekens, C., Willett, W.C., et al. "Prospective

study of nutritional factors, blood pressure, and hypertension among U.S. women." *Hypertension*, 1996;27:1065–72.

5. Reyes, A.J., Leary, W.P. "Cardiovascular toxicity of diuretics related to magnesium depletion." *Human Toxicology*, 1984;3(5):351–71.

6. Cohen, J.S. "Adverse drug effects, compliance, and the initial doses of antihypertensive drugs recommended by the Joint National Community vs. the *Physicians' Desk Reference*." *Archives of Internal Medicine*, March 26, 2001;161:880–85.

7. Cohen, J.S. "Dose Discrepancies between the *Physicians' Desk Reference* and the Medical Literature, and Their Possible Role in the High Incidence of Dose-Related Adverse Drug Events." *Archives of Internal Medicine*, April 9, 2001:161:957–64.

8. Cohen, J.S. "Do Standard Doses of Frequently Prescribed Drugs Cause Preventable Adverse Effects in Women?" *JAMWA (The Journal of the American Medical Women's Association)*, 2002;57:105–110.

9. Cohen, J.S. *Over Dose: The Case Against The Drug Companies. Prescription Drugs, Side Effects, and Your Health.* Tarcher/Putnam, New York: October 2001.

10. Resnick, L.M., Bardicef, O., Altura, B.T., Alderman, M.H., and Altura, B.M. "Serum ionized magnesium: relation to blood pressure and racial factors." *American Journal of Hypertension*, 1997;10(12 Pt 1):1420–4.

11. Ma, J., Folsom, A.R., et al. "Associations of serum and dietary magnesium with cardiovascular disease, hypertension, diabetes, insulin, and carotid arterial wall thickness: the ARIC study. Atherosclerosis Risk in Communities Study." *Journal of Clinical Epidemiology*, 1995;48(7):927–40.

12. Bakris, G.L. "A Practical Approach to Achieving Recommended Blood Pressure Goals in Diabetic Patients." *Archives of Internal Medicine*, 2001;161:2661–67.

13. Villarosa, L. "A New Message Emerges in Treating Diabetes." *New York Times*, 9/2/03:nytimes.com.

14. Bloomgarden, Z.T. "American Diabetes Association scientific sessions, 1995. Magnesium deficiency, atherosclerosis, and health care." *Diabetes Care*, 1995;18(12):1623–7.

15. Resnick, L.M. "Magnesium in the Pathophysiology and Treatment of Hypertension and Diabetes Mellitus: Where Are We in 1997?" *American Journal of Hypertension,* 1997;10(3): 368–70.

16. Kawano Y., Matsuoka, H., Takishita, S., and Omae, T. "Effects of magnesium supplementation in hypertensive patients: assessment by office, home, and ambulatory blood pressures." *Hypertension,* 1998;32:260–265.

17. Altura, B.M., and Altura, B.T. "Magnesium in Cardiovascular Biology." *Scientific American,* Science & Medicine, May/June 1995:28–37.

18. Logan, AG. "The DASH trials implicate dysfunction in calcium regulation in the pathogenesis of human hypertension." *Current Hypertension Reports,* 2001;3(5):367–70.

19. Altura, B.M., and Altura, B.T. "Magnesium in Cardiovascular Biology." *Scientific American,* Science & Medicine, May/June 1995:28–37.

20. Paolisso, G., and Barbagallo, M. "Hypertension, diabetes mellitus, and insulin resistance: the role of intracellular magnesium." *American Journal of Hypertension,* 1997;10(3):346–55.

21. Lima de, L.M., Cruz, T., Pousada, J.C., et al. "The effect of magnesium supplementation in increasing doses on the control of type 2 diabetes." *Diabetes Care,* 1998;21(5):682–6.

22. Resnick, L.M. "Magnesium in the Pathophysiology and Treatment of Hypertension and Diabetes Mellitus: Where Are We in 1997?" *American Journal of Hypertension,* 1997;10(3):368–70.

23. Izzo, J.L., and Black, H.R. "Hypertension Primer: The Essentials of High Blood Pressure." *American Heart Association,* Dallas: 1999.

24. Kaplan, N.M. "Hypertension in the Population at Large." Chapter 1 in *Clinical Hypertension.* Baltimore: Williams and Wilkins, 1998.

25. Izzo, J.L., and Black, H.R. "Hypertension Primer: The Essentials of High Blood Pressure." *American Heart Association,* Dallas: 1999.

26. Kisters, K., Schodjaian, K., Tokmak, F., et al. "Effect of ethanol on blood pressure—role of magnesium [letter]." *American Journal of Hypertension,* 2000;13(4 Pt 1):455–6.

4. How to Use Magnesium to Help Prevent and Treat Hypertension

1. Magaziner, A. Personal communications, Nov. 28, 2001 and Dec. 2, 2001.

2. Whitaker, J. "Fortify Yourself with the Most Important—and Most Overlooked—Supplement of All." *Health & Healing*, Mid-August 1992;2(9):1.

3. "The Sixth Report of the Joint National Committee on Prevention, Detection, Evaluation, and Treatment of High Blood Pressure." *Archives of Internal Medicine*, 1997;157:2413–46.

4. Appel, L.J., Moore, T.J., Obarzanek, E., Vollmer, W.M., Svetkey, L.P., Sacks, F.M., et al. "A clinical trial of the effects of dietary patterns on blood pressure. DASH Collaborative Research Group." *New England Journal of Medicine*, 1997;336(16):1117–24.

5. "The Sixth Report of the Joint National Committee on Prevention, Detection, Evaluation, and Treatment of High Blood Pressure." *Archives of Internal Medicine*, 1997;157:2413–46.

6. Laurant, P., and Touyz, R.M. "Physiological and pathophysiological role of magnesium in the cardiovascular system: implications in hypertension." *Journal of Hypertension*, 2000;18(9): 1177–91.

7. Whitaker, J. "Minerals, Part 2: Miraculous Magnesium." *Health and Healing*, May 1999;9(5):2.

8. Whitaker, J. "The Three Minerals That Control Your Blood Pressure." *Health and Healing*, Mar. 1994; 4:3.

9. Mende, C. Personal communication, Sept. 25, 2001.

10. Kaplan, N.M. "Hypertension in the Population at Large." Chapter 1 in *Clinical Hypertension*. Baltimore: Williams and Wilkins, 1998.

11. Magaziner, A. Personal communications, Nov. 28, 2001 and Dec. 2, 2001.

12. Whitaker, J. "Minerals, Part 2: Miraculous Magnesium." *Health and Healing*, May 1999;9(5):2.

13. Seelig, M.S., Rosanoff, A. *The magnesium factor*. New York: Penguin Group Inc. 2003.

14. Magaziner, A. Personal communications, Nov. 28, 2001 and Dec. 2, 2001.

15. ALLHAT Collaborative Research Group. "Major Outcomes in High-Risk Hypertensive Patients Randomized to Angiotensin-Converting Enzyme Inhibitor or Calcium Channel Blocker vs Diuretic: The Antihypertensive and Lipid-Lowering Treatment to Prevent Heart Attack Trial (ALLHAT)." *JAMA*, 2002;288:2981–2997.

16. Reyes, A.J., and Alcocer, L. "Minding Magnesium While Treating Essential Hypertension with Diuretics." In: Theophanides, T., and Anastassopoulou, J. *Magnesium: current status and new developments.* Dordrecht [Netherlands]: Kluwer Academic, 1997.

17. Mende, C. Personal communication, Sept. 25, 2001.

18. Sheehan, J.P., and Seelig, M.S. "Interactions of magnesium and potassium in the pathogenesis of cardiovascular disease." *Magnesium*, 1984;3(4–6):301–14.

19. Ascherio, A., Hennekens, C., Willett, W.C., et al. "Prospective study of nutritional factors, blood pressure, and hypertension among U.S. women." *Hypertension*, 1996;27:1065–72.

20. Cohen, E., Wheat, M.E., Swiderski, D.M., and Charney, P. "Hypertension in Women." Chapter 11 in Laragh, J.H., Brenner, B.M., *Hypertension: Pathophysiology, Diagnosis, and Management.* Second Edition. New York: Raven Press Limited, 1995.

21. Logan, A.G. "The DASH trials implicate dysfunction in calcium regulation in the pathogenesis of human hypertension." *Current Hypertension Reports*, 2001;3(5):367–70.

22. Elson, B.D. Personal communication, Nov. 28, 2001.

23. "The Sixth Report of the Joint National Committee on Prevention, Detection, Evaluation, and Treatment of High Blood Pressure." *Archives of Internal Medicine*, 1997;157:2413–46.

24. Logan, A.G. "The DASH trials implicate dysfunction in calcium regulation in the pathogenesis of human hypertension." *Current Hypertension Reports*, 2001;3(5):367–70.

25. Laurant, P., and Touyz, R.M. "Physiological and pathophysiological role of magnesium in the cardiovascular system: implications in hypertension." *Journal of Hypertension*, 2000;18(9):1177–91.

26. Sacks, F.M., Svetkey, L.P., Vollmer, W.M., et al. "Effects on blood pressure of reduced dietary sodium and the Dietary Approaches to Stop Hypertension (DASH) diet. DASH-Sodium Collaborative Research Group." *New England Journal of Medicine*, 2001;344(1):3–10.

27. Conlin, P.R., Chow, D., Miller, E.R. 3rd, et al. "The effect of dietary patterns on blood pressure control in hypertensive patients: results from the Dietary Approaches to Stop Hypertension (DASH) trial." *American Journal of Hypertension*, 2000;13(9):949–55.

28. Van Leer, E.M., Seidell, J.C., and Kromhout, D. "Dietary calcium, potassium, magnesium and blood pressure in the Netherlands." *International Journal of Epidemiology*, 1995;24(6):1117–23.

29. Resnick, L.M. "Magnesium in the Pathophysiology and Treatment of Hypertension and Diabetes Mellitus: Where Are We in 1997?" *American Journal of Hypertension*, 1997;10(3): 368–70.

30. "The Sixth Report of the Joint National Committee on Prevention, Detection, Evaluation, and Treatment of High Blood Pressure." *Archives of Internal Medicine*, 1997;157:2413–46.

31. Whitaker, J. "Minerals, Part 2: Miraculous Magnesium." *Health and Healing*, May 1999;9(5):2.

32. Karppanen, H., Tanskanen, A., Tuomilehto, J., et al. "Safety and effects of potassium- and magnesium-containing low sodium salt mixtures." *Journal of Cardiovascular Pharmacology*, 1984;6 (Suppl 1):S236–43.

33. Katz, A., Rosenthal, T., Maoz, C., et al. "Effect of a mineral salt diet on 24-h blood pressure monitoring in elderly hypertensive patients." *Journal of Human Hypertension*, 1999;13(11):777–80.

34. Geleijnse, J.M., Witteman, J.C., Bak, A.A., et al. "Reduction in blood pressure with a low sodium, high potassium, high magnesium salt in older subjects with mild to moderate hypertension." *BMJ*, 1994;309(6952):436–40.

ABOUT THE AUTHOR

Dr. Jay Cohen is a widely recognized expert on prescription medications and non-drug alternatives that work. Dr. Cohen is an Associate Professor (voluntary) of Family and Preventive Medicine and of Psychiatry at the University of California, San Diego. Dr. Cohen graduated from Temple University School of Medicine in Philadelphia in 1971. After completing his internship, Dr. Cohen practiced general medicine, then conducted pain research at UCLA. He then completed a psychiatry residency at the University of California, San Diego, and practiced psychiatry and psychopharmacology for thirteen years.

Since 1990, Dr. Cohen has been involved in clinical pharmacology, conducting independent research on medication side effects: why they occur and how they can be prevented. Dr. Cohen's research has identified multiple problems—in drug industry research, U.S. Food and Drug Administration review, and doctors' methods—that have contributed to medication side effects being the fourth leading cause of death in America. Dr. Cohen believes that most medication side effects are preventable.

Since 1996, Dr. Cohen has published his findings and solutions in leading medical journals including the *Archives of Internal Medicine, The Journal of the American Medical Women's Association, Geriatrics, Drug Safety, and the Annals of Pharmacotherapy*. He has also written articles for consumer publications such as *Newsweek, Bottom Line Health,* and *Life Extension Magazine.* His work has been featured in the *New York Times, Washington Post, Consumer Reports, Wall Street Journal, Modern Maturity, Women's Day,* and virtually every other major magazine and newspaper in America. His book, *Over Dose: The Case Against The Drug Companies* (Tarcher/Putnam, Nov. 2001), received unanimously excellent reviews from Publishers Weekly, Library Journal, and others, as well as from the *Journal of the American Medical Association.*

Dr. Cohen has been featured on more than 75 radio programs across America including National Public Radio. Dr. Cohen has spoken at conferences conducted for patients, doctors, drug industry executives, and malpractice attorneys. In October 2001, during the anthrax scare, Dr. Cohen's article on severe reactions to Cipro Levaquin and other fluoroquinolone antibiotics triggered a national debate on the best treatment for anthrax and prompted the U.S. Centers for Disease Control to alter their treatment guidelines. In November 2002, Dr. Cohen was the keynote speaker at the Annual Science Day of the U.S. Food and Drug Administration's Clinical Pharmacology Division.

In September 2003, the author created the Center for the Prevention of Medication Side Effects, a non-profit (tax-exempt status pending) corporation to support his work. Through its website (www.MedicationSense.com) and free electronic newsletter, the Center provides free, independent information to patients and healthcare professionals on strategies for maximizing the benefits while minimizing the risks of prescription and over-the-counter drugs as well as supplements and other natural therapies. The Center and its MedicationSense.com website offers information about drugs, doses, and side effects, which is not available in mainstream sources or standard drug references.

Dr. Cohen emphasizes that patients have a right to informed consent about medications. Informed consent requires full knowledge of the lowest, safest, effective doses of drugs. Today, such information is frequently omitted from package inserts and drug references used by doctors and patients. Informed consent should also include information about natural substances which, like magnesium, are proven effective in scientific studies. The mission of the Center for the Prevention of Medication Side Effects is to research and communicate these issues with clear, practical guidelines that will enable patients to obtain the most effective treatments with the least risks. For more information, go to www.MedicationSense.com.

INDEX

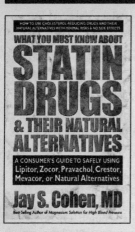

WHAT YOU MUST KNOW ABOUT STATIN DRUGS & THEIR NATURAL ALTERNATIVES
A Consumer's Guide to Safely Using Lipitor, Zocor, Pravachol, Crestor, Mevacor, or Natural Alternatives

Jay S. Cohen, MD

It is estimated that over 100 million Americans suffer from elevated cholesterol and C-reactive proteins—markers that are linked to heart attack, stroke, and other cardiovascular disorders. To combat these problems, modern science has created a group of drugs known either as statins or as specific commercial drugs such as Lipitor, Zocor, and Pravachol. While over 20 million people take these medications, the fact is that up to 42 percent experience side effects, and a whopping 60 to 70 percent eventually stop treatment. Here, for the first time, is a guide that explains the problems caused by statins, and offers easy-to-follow strategies that will allow you to benefit from these drugs while avoiding their side effects. In addition, the author provides natural alternatives that have also proven effective.

What You Must Know About Statin Drugs & Their Natural Alternatives begins by explaining elevated cholesterol and C-reactive proteins. It then examines how statins work to alleviate these problems, and discusses possible side effects. Highlighted is information on safe usage, as well as a discussion of effective alternative treatments. If you have elevated cholesterol and C-reactive proteins, or if you are currently using a statin, *What You Must Know About Statin Drugs & Their Natural Alternatives* can make a profound difference in the quality of your life.

$14.95 • 204 pages • 6 x 9-inch paperback • Health • ISBN 0-7570-0257-9

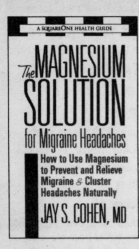